MRCP

Clinical Examination

A PRACTICAL GUIDE

- Communication Scenarios
- Clinical Stations
- Development
- History Taking and Management Planning
- Video Scenarios
- Online Video Links

Overcoming the Challenges of the
MRCPCH Clinical Examination

Abbreviations

Abbreviations	Full form
ICS	Inter costal spaces
BP	Blood pressure
CBT	Cognitive behaviour therapy
MRI	Magnetic resonance imaging
IQ	Intelligent quotient
TSC	Tuberous sclerosis complex
DLA	Disability living allowance
OPD	Out Patient Department
PEFR	Peak expiratory flow rate
SALT	Speech and Language Therapy

MRCPCH
Clinical Examination

A PRACTICAL GUIDE

- Communication Scenarios
- Clinical Stations
- Development
- History Taking and Management Planning
- Video Scenarios
- Online Video Links

Anil Garg

FRCPCH, FRCPI, DCH, Dip. Educ. PG Cert. Medical Careers

Consultant Paediatrician, Western Sussex Hospitals NHS Trust
Principal Regional Examiner, Royal College of Paediatrics and Child Health
Honarary Consultant Paediatrician, Brighton Sussex University Hospitals NHS Trust
Associate Professor, American University of Caribbean, St Marteen

Siba Prosad Paul

MBBS, DCH, MRCPCH

ST4 in Paediatrics, St. Richard's Hospital
Speciality Trainee in Paediatrics, Severn Deanery (UK)
Chichester, UK

CBS

CBS Publishers & Distributors Pvt Ltd

New Delhi • Bengaluru • Pune • Kochi • Chennai
Mumbai • Kolkata • Hyderabad • Patna • Manipal

MRCPCH
Clinical Examination
A PRACTICAL GUIDE

ISBN: 978-81-239-2238-6

Copyright © Authors and Publisher

First Edition: 2013

Published by Satish Kumar Jain and produced by Vinod K. Jain for

CBS Publishers & Distributors Pvt Ltd
4819/XI Prahlad Street, 24 Ansari Road, Daryaganj, New Delhi 110 002, India.
Ph: 23289259, 23266861, 23266867

Fax: 011-23243014

Website: www.cbspd.com
e-mail: delhi@cbspd.com; cbspubs@airtelmail.in

Corporate Office: 204 FIE, Industrial Area, Patparganj, Delhi 110 092
Ph: 4934 4934

Fax: 4934 4935

e-mail: publishing@cbspd.com; publicity@cbspd.com

Branches

- **Bengaluru:** Seema House 2975, 17th Cross, K.R. Road,
  Banasankari 2nd Stage, Bengaluru 560 070, Karnataka
  Ph: +91-80-26771678/79　　　Fax: +91-80-26771680　　e-mail: bangalore@cbspd.com
- **Pune:** Bhuruk Prestige, Sr. No. 52/12/2+1+3/2 Narhe, Haveli
  (Near Katraj-Dehu Road Bypass), Pune 411 041, Maharashtra
  Ph: +91-20-64704058, 64704059, 32342277　　Fax: +91-20-24300160　　e-mail: pune@cbspd.com
- **Kochi:** 36/14 Kalluvilakam, Lissie Hospital Road, Kochi 682 018, Kerala
  Ph: +91-484-4059061-65　　　Fax: +91-484-4059065　　e-mail: cochin@cbspd.com
- **Chennai:** 20, West Park Road, Shenoy Nagar, Chennai 600 030, Tamil Nadu
  Ph: +91-44-26260666, 26208620　　Fax: +91-44-45530020　　e-mail: chennai@cbspd.com

Representatives

- **Mumbai**　0-9833017933
- **Patna**　0-9334159340
- **Kolkata**　0-9831437309
- **Manipal**　0-9742022075
- **Hyderabad**　0-9885175004

Printed at Manipal Technologies Limited, Manipal

The Royal Colleges in the United Kingdom have a unique history of assessing the postgraduate medical trainee in a fair and rigorous manner. This is appreciated and valued by the trainees. There is thus a great demand for being assessed by this process among postgraduate trainees in paediatrics in South Asia and other parts of the world. There is substantial personal satisfaction in being approved by the process, and obtaining the MRCPCH is an important landmark in the career trajectory of many paediatricians.

The consumers in South Asia also hold similar views. I have come across many grandparents and young parents in cities such as Kolkata actively looking for "a paediatrician with an MRCPCH" for the management of their ill child or grandchild. I have often wondered why this is the case, in a country which has many excellent institutions for teaching medicine at both under- and postgraduate levels.

The truth is that within a healthcare system that is largely 'private' and less closely regulated as is the case in India and other countries in South Asia, the RCPCH continues to provide a robust and scrupulously fair system of postgraduate assessment in paediatrics that leads in the end to a hallmark of quality for the candidate who successfully qualifies for his MRCPCH. It is remarkable how the consumers, the parents of young children, in cities such as Kolkata and Mumbai, respect this, and continue to place their trust in the judgement of the RCPCH assessors and in the judgement of the assessment system developed by the RCPCH. Many large hospitals in India that have helped revolutionise healthcare in recent times also place considerable reliance on the training and assessment programme of the RCPCH in the choice of their medical staff.

The RCPCH and its assessors are thus in effect involved in a long-term, close, collaborative and enormously fruitful and important partnership with the people and many of the health care providers in India and other countries in South Asia.

This book is a culmination of a number of aspects of this process of collaboration, and represents an important milestone within this development. There has been a need for systematic step-by-step guidance for postgraduate trainees in paediatrics aspiring for the MRCPCH. There is also a need for this guidance to be carefully tailored to the needs of postgraduate trainees in paediatrics from Asia. Anil Garg and Siba Paul's excellent book and accompanying web resource aims to provide this guidance. I am delighted to support the development of this important programme that is likely to benefit a generation of postgraduate paediatric trainees worldwide.

Professor Somnath Mukhopadhyay
MBBS (Kolkata, India, 1983) MD PhD FRCPCH
Chair of Paediatrics
Royal Alexandra Children's Hospital
Brighton and Sussex Medical School
Eastern Road, Brighton, BN2 5BE
United Kingdom

Foreword

MRCPCH is essentially an examination for the paediatric trainees in the UK. However, over the years it has become one of the most prestigious paediatric examinations with high international reputation. The status of this examination emanates from the fact that huge amount of work goes in to ensuring that the examination is based on solid principles, the assessment is fair and discriminatory. All stages of the examination are evaluated rigorously and continuously. I frequently hear the comments that having taken the examination one is a better paediatrician. This is a tribute to the quality of this examination.

I am delighted that the MRCPCH examination is now available to be taken in India. This is a great opportunity for trainees in India who do not have to travel to UK and can acquire an international qualification which will boost their career prospects in India and abroad.

Dr Anil Garg is an esteemed colleague of high reputation in UK. It is obvious that the authors have experience of working in India as well UK which is reflected in the style of presentation. It is written in simple, easy to understand language with excellent practical advice to candidates who have not worked in UK. The notes at the end of each scenario are evidence-based and referenced when required. I very much liked "Remember !" the invaluable tips in passing the examination. I thoroughly enjoyed reading the book and learnt a few things myself.

I hope this book will assist you not only in passing the examination but also in being a good paediatrician. I congratulate the authors for a quality book which I am sure will be of immense value to those taking the clinical examination.

Dr Ramesh Mehta FRCPCH, FRCP, MD, DCH, FHEA
Senior Examiner and Consultant Paediatrician
Bedford Hospital, UK
Vice Chair, RCPCH, UK

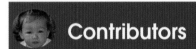 # Contributors

Anil Garg MBBS, DCH, FRCPCH, FRCPI, Dip.Edu.
Consultant Paediatrician, Western Sussex Hospitals NHS Trust
Principal Regional Examiner, Royal College of Paediatrics and Child Health
Honorary Consultant Paediatrician, Brighton Sussex University Hospitals NHS Trust
Associate Clinical Professor, American University of Caribbean, St Marteen

Siba Prosad Paul MBBS, DCH, MRCPCH
ST4 in Paediatrics, St Richard's Hospital, Chichester, UK

Sujata Edate MBBS, DCH, DNB, MRCPCH
ST6 in Paediatrics, St Peter's Hospital, Chertsey

Dinakaran Rengan MBBS, MD, MRCPCH
ST4 in Paediatrics, St. Richard's Hospital, Chichester

Nirajan Mukherjee MBBS, DCH, MRCPCH
ST5 in Paediatrics, King's College Hospital, London

Urmila Pillai MBBS, DCH, MD, DNB, MRCPCH
Assistant Professor, BC Roy Memorial Children's Hospital, Kolkata

Royal College of Paediatrics and Child Health (RCPCH) is responsible for the training and examination of paediatricians in the United Kingdom. Membership of the RCPCH (MRCPCH) is achieved after rigorous training and examination. It is achieved by passing 3 sets of examinations. The first two are written examinations that test the knowledge of paediatrics—theoretical (MRCPCH 1 A & B) and applied (MRCPCH 2 written). These are followed by the MRCPCH Part II Clinical: The final hurdle!

The MRCPCH examination is a good tool to assess whether you (the candidate) are ready to take the next step in your career of a more senior paediatrician. This exam is aimed at testing your knowledge of paediatrics and also expects you to demonstrate that you apply this knowledge in the clinical practice. This needs practice and above all ability to demonstrate that before the examiners in a controlled environment. Please be courteous and kind to the children and their family, they are there for your benefit on the day, having left aside their daily schedule.

Success in the MRCPCH signifies that the holder has achieved breadth and depth of knowledge in paediatrics to a high degree. The success also signifies that the doctor has demonstrated their ability to apply this knowledge in the clinical context, therefore, can be trusted to care for sick children.

This book is aimed at preparing you and explains what to expect on the day. In the exam how an OSCE (objective structured clinical examination) is conducted and useful tips that (we as authors feel) will help you in achieving what you have been working for the MRCPCH of the RCPCH, UK. This book is intended to sharpen your observation and presentation skills and to bring out the knowledge you have and have demonstrated by having passed the written exams.

MRCPCH being primarily a UK based examination, it is possible that paediatricians preparing for the exam overseas may not be acquainted with multidisciplinary approach taken towards management of chronic conditions and safeguarding of children. The book will, therefore, highlight on such aspects that may not form part of everyday paediatric practice while working overseas. Some aspects highlighted will be child protection, breaking bad news, dealing with a difficult colleague, managing chronic conditions (diabetes, asthma, and others), and expectation to work in a multidisciplinary team. These themes are often assessed in the clinical exam and every candidate will have to encounter these in some form, be it a communication scenario, history taking or a part of answering the questions in a clinical examination station.

This book will be particularly helpful to the paediatricians working overseas and preparing to take the exam at an overseas location or visiting the UK with the purpose of appearing in the MRCPCH clinical exam. The book is equally relevant for doctors working in the UK in their preparation for the exam.

We have endeavoured to provide guidance on the aspects mentioned above in addition to highlighting commonly encountered clinical stations in the exam that candidates find more difficult. Useful tips are provided in a box to highlight the learning opportunity that can make a difference to your performance.

We have incorporated pictures in the book to give examples of the condition and some relevant clinical points. The information is not aimed to be comprehensive as there are a number of text and reference books in paediatrics but to highlight points for possible discussion and reflection. It will be important to study them as you may encounter the 'condition' in different parts of the examination, i.e. video station or written Part 2.

Some model communication scenarios and history taking and discussion are available to give a flair of as how to these may be approached in the examination. These are available on a disk or on line.

There are many ways of reaching the goal and ours is only one of them. Working through this book will give you an advantage with your preparation and performance for that final day.

We are open to your comments and value the suggestions for improving this book or its contents in the future.

The 'golden mantra' is "good focused preparation" and "failing to prepare is preparing to fail." So ... 'Practice!, Practice!, Practice!'

We hope you enjoy reading the book and all the best for the exam.

Anil Garg

docgargs@gmail.com

Siba Prosad Paul

siba_prosad@yahoo.co.uk

Contents

Introduction to Clinical Examination

Communication

Clinical Stations

Development

Focused History and Management Planning

Video Station

Appendices

Introduction to
Clinical Examination

The RCPCH came into existence in 1996 by Royal charter, separating from the Royal College of Physicians. The MRCPCH examination succeeded MRCP (paediatrics) that was conferred by the Royal College of Physicians earlier. The new format of the MRCPCH clinical examination was piloted in 2004 and is considered to be fairer to the candidates, more robust and reproducible. It has Objective Structured Clinical Examination (OSCE) format and tests competencies that a postgraduate professional needs.

The exam has a total of 10 stations: 6 clinical examination stations, 2 communication stations, 1 history and management and 1 video station. The video station will have 8 to 10 video topics to test on your management of paediatric conditions that are crucial to the paediatric training and clinical practice but may not be suitable to be tested in clinical examination setting.

RCPCH invests great effort in ensuring every exam is thorough, fair and of comparable standard to previous exams. The written questions and video scenarios are prepared and checked in different settings before being included in an exam. Candidate response is monitored to judge reliability, ease and discriminatory power to each question. In the clinical exams, a summary of the 'child's' illness with details of clinical signs is available to the examiners. However, each child is examined by 2 examiners before each session, to confirm the signs that are used to standard set for the ensuing session.

Figure below highlights the circuit that will be encountered on the day of the exam and further details are available at the College website www.rcpch.ac.uk

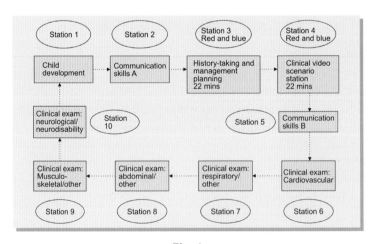

Fig. 1

During the examination 'circuit', a candidate spends 9 minutes at each clinical station. 12 candidates start together – 6 at clinical stations, 2 at communication stations, 2 at history-taking and management station and 2 at video stations.

Each clinical station lasts 13 minutes: 9 minutes are spent with the patient and examiner and 4 minutes are spent in between stations. The candidate is invited into the room at the ring of a bell. Examiner will greet the candidate, take the mark sheet, introduce the patient and define the specific task. The candidate will not be interrupted, at 7 minutes there is a knock to mark 2 minutes remain. It is expected the candidate will have completed the given task, they will be asked to summarize the case and a discussion with the examiner will follow. A bell sounds at 9 minutes when the candidate leaves the room. The candidate will then move to the next station and wait for approximately 4 minutes when the bell rings again and the cycle starts.

During the 4 minutes while the candidate waits outside and prepares for the next station, the examiner will decide on the performance on the station just completed. This is done against the standards that has been set for the patient before the beginning of the exam by two examiners, who have examined the patient together. The mark sheet is completed by the examiner and comments are written about performance for later feedback.

The statements specific tasks for a clinical examination could be
1. "Please examine John's chest, he is a 6-year-old, referred by his General Practitioner with recurrent chest infections".
2. "Please examine Abdul, 5-year-old, who has been noted to have a murmur at a routine consultation for fever".
3. "Please examine Susan's legs, her mother is worried about her walking with a limp".

History-taking and management and video stations last 22 minutes at the end of which the candidate leaves the room and moves on to the next station and waits for approximately 4 minutes – total 26 minutes.

Paediatric Training in UK

The paediatric training in the UK is spread over a 8-year period (ST 1–8) and is delivered by a 2 tier system: the junior trainees receives training for 3 years and are expected to achieve a certain standard to get into the middle grade tier. Success in the MRCPCH examination is the necessary benchmark for a trainee to be considered ready to take up a more senior role with Consultant supervision. This concept has been nicely demonstrated in the Miller's pyramid which maps the different methods of assessment the MRCPCH exam aims at and also how a paediatrician in training works through the system to become a consultant in the UK.

MRCPCH exam has international recognition: this signifies that the 'holder' has achieved a 'high level' of competence in the field of child health and therefore

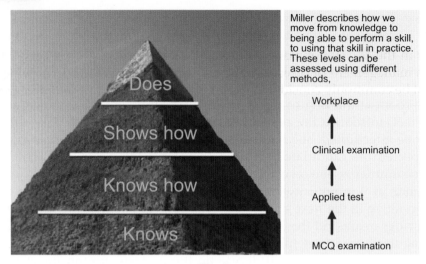

Miller describes how we move from knowledge to being able to perform a skill, to using that skill in practice. These levels can be assessed using different methods,

Does

Shows how

Knows how

Knows

Workplace

↑

Clinical examination

↑

Applied test

↑

MCQ examination

Fig. 2

can be trusted with the care of a sick child. Paediatricians are essential in improving the care for children. The MRCPCH exam has been extended to other countries over the years to assist with training of paediatricians abroad. It is recognized as a postgraduate paediatric qualification in Singapore, Hong Kong, Egypt, UAE, Kuwait, Bahrain, Oman and list is growing. The MRCPCH has been more recently introduced in India and is being conducted in 5 centers: Bengaluru, Chennai, Delhi, Kolkata and Mumbai. This enables the candidate to sit the exam in India and to avoid need of travel to the UK.

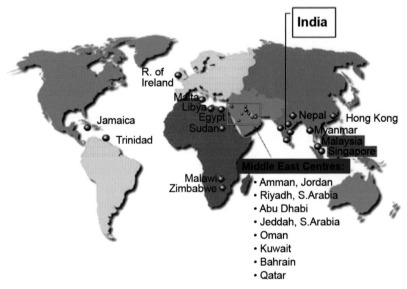

India

R. of Ireland

Malta
Libya
Egypt
Sudan

Jamaica

Trinidad

Nepal   Hong Kong
Myanmar
Malaysia
Singapore

Malawi
Zimbabwe

Middle East Centres:
• Amman, Jordan
• Riyadh, S.Arabia
• Abu Dhabi
• Jeddah, S.Arabia
• Oman
• Kuwait
• Bahrain
• Qatar

Fig. 3

The MRCPCH examination tests areas that are important in good care of a sick child as well as a child with a chronic condition by involving the child and parents in the decision making process, a practice that in not universal. It also tests on management of disease in the UK setting. It thus tests areas which that may not be commonly considered essential or practiced by a paediatrician while in training at an overseas hospital.

Some adjustments are expected to be made in the clinical examination format to meet the local disease prevalence, needs of children and examinees appearing in the MRCPCH exam overseas. However, it needs to be remembered that this is primarily an UK exam and some knowledge of how paediatrics is practiced in the UK will be necessary to meet the standards of the examination.

We highlight areas that have been noted to cause 'difficulty' to candidates leading to a performance which the candidate may consider has been marked below par to their expectation. Our experience is that with proper guidance and practice, the candidates can improve their performance during the examination and have better chances of achieving success in the MRCPCH.

Your preparation for the exam begins before you get to the exam centre. On the day dress in a conservative style and present a professional image. On the way to the exam centre stay calm and do not get worked up. Ensure you get there in good time as any delay or potential delays will only increase tension and your ability to perform well on this most significant day. Check out the route and get a good nights rest.

Examination is a very artificial situation, it is not only about what you know but you have to 'show' what you know. You have to 'perform' and show off your different skills and competences that will be tested, history-taking and management discussion, communications with patients, parents, medical students, nurses and other colleagues, system examinations: cardiovascular, neurology, development, respiratory, abdomen and other.

We all find 'Being observed and being monitored' a very uncomfortable experience. During our routine work activities, our clerking and clinical findings are ratified by our seniors and peers but we are never really 'observed' while getting that information. In a survey in my hospital a few years ago most doctors had only been 'observed' during their undergraduate medical exam and then in their postgraduate membership exam.

Thus to 'ignore' you are being observed and 'perform' as normal, you will need to practice. Ask your colleagues to observe you and give feedback on your performance.

Current trainees in UK undergo workplace based assessments that prepare them to 'perform' while being observed. Ask to be observed while taking a history or examining and get feedback.

During the examination you will have to present your finding a number of times. I suggest you use the 4-point presentation as this will keep you in control and lead to logical discussion where you will score the extra marks.

- **General findings on observation**
- **Important positive finding**
- **Important relevant negative finding**
- **Overall conclusion**

This will usually be followed by discussing on investigations, treatment options, explaining disease processes or relevant ethical issues, e.g.

- **General findings**
  I have seen, X, a 8-year-old boy who is comfortable and pink at rest (*mention any drugs or medical devices that you can see, i.e. inhaler devices, wheel chair, splints,*

oxygen cylinder, medication, protective head gear). If there is nothings, it is worth mentioning the absence of any special equipment.

- **Important positive findings**
  I note he looks rather small for his age, would like to plot his height and weight on an appropriate chart, he has a 'portcath' on the left side of his chest, otherwise chest is symmetrical with equal expansion, there is equal air entry and normal breath sound.
  I note he has a large number of drugs – specific names if possible (*can lead to diagnosis of cystic fibrosis in a child with 'normal' examination*) and sputum pot on the side table.

- **Important relevant negative findings**
  There is no clubbing, no cyanosis and there are no other scars on his chest.

- **Overall conclusion**
  The features are suggestive of a chronic condition. The most likely diagnosis in view of the medications and portacath being cystic fibrosis, he is comparatively well controlled and there are no stigmata of the disease.

From here on the discussion will follow and you should be prepared. You should know cystic fibrosis in detail as the discussion will be more important and extensive as there were minimal clinical findings.

In the above example the diagnosis is certain but otherwise you need to be prepared with a differential diagnosis – top 3 conditions.

Answering a Question

You will be replying to questions all through the exam. It is important to think through a strategy that will guide you through most situations and keep you in control of the situation.

- Do not be tempted to reply/speak immediately.
- Do not say the first thing that comes to mind – hoping others ideas will follow.
- Take up to 10 seconds to think over the question carefully.
- Work out what is being asked, try to differentiate from what you think you heard.
- Think of 3 common points in relation to the question asked.
- If possible, think of the next question to follow on from your answer.
- With practice – this is all possible.
- When you do start reply – keep your thoughts 5 seconds ahead of your mouth.

You may think the initial silence will be awkward, the first 5–10 seconds may seem like 'eternity' but believe me, a 10 second gap half-way through your answer, when you do not know what to say, will be a lot more awkward and 'deafening' than the first pause.

If you are *not* sure of what is being asked – CLARIFY.

"How would you mange her VSD?" "Am I being asked about how to manage changes to the management?" It is better than going down the wrong path, wasting your valuable time and not scoring any marks. Here you will be expected to talk about symptom management, medications, and medium to longer term plan, including possible need for surgery and discussion with parents – *not* about pathophysiology of VSD.

When you do start answering 'guide' the examiner to areas you know well. If talking about differential diagnosis - stick to three common ones. If it so happens you feel you do not know enough about a particular condition *do not* mention it, as long as it is not the first on the list. If it happens that you do not know details and are not in a position to discuss—then admit your lack of knowledge and the discussion will move on—you will continue to earn marks. *Do not* bluff as that is easily noted by experienced examiners.

When speaking to 'parents' or 'patients' in exam setting – always check their understanding first.

"What have you been told so far?" or "What do you understand is the matter with your son/daughter?" "What are you most concerned about?" Here also follow the above strategy and be prepared to say "I do *not* know enough to tell you but I will find out and come back and let you know".

You may feel reading the repeated emphasis on communication as an 'overkill' but the time you spend now on practicing and improving this skill will help you more than anything else you may do so close to the exam.

Communication

Communication

Communication is fundamental to our interaction with other people. We communicate our thoughts by a number of ways: the spoken word, written word, with gestures, eye contact, our body with its own body language and with pictures and diagrams. We use all of the various methods of communication mentioned without being aware and move from one to the other seamlessly. Research has shown that majority of our communication is nonverbal. Our speech and tone of our voice play a significant role hence be aware of these as they have greater impact than what you actually say.

You should use spoken words most of the time but be aware of relevance of written words and diagrams as also a very effective way of getting your message across.

Three Way Consultation

In paediatrics, our patient is a child and the carer / 'worriers' are the parents. We have to develop skills to be able to engage both appropriately. It is always important to interact with the child and include them in the discussion as much as possible. **You ignore the child at your peril and will be marked down if you fail to engage the child.** If a child is present, start by interacting with the child with an opening remark of welcoming them or introducing yourself and a question they should be able to answer. "What did you do at school yesterday or what do you like at school best." You can them move on to indirect and direct questions to gain the information: "What games do you play? If you had a race in your class where will you come? Can you play like your friends or do you get out of 'puff' and have to stop?" No point asking "How much exercise you can do?" The parents can then be asked to fill in other relevant information or correct information they feel needs amending. At the end of the consultation – make sure you let the child know – in simpler language what you would like them to do and thank them.

Communication station is not a knowledge testing exercise. You **do not have to show how much you know of a particular condition**. It is about how you engage with the person, develop a two way dialogue, elicit and address their concerns and give what information they need, in a language and manner they can understand. Try and establish what they know already, make a judgement of their level of understanding and pitch your message at appropriate level. You may ask what they do and the language of your answer should be different, though not its content, if you were speaking to a cleaner versus a physics teacher in secondary school when explaining about say a murmur. **My suggestion will** be to start with as if you were talking to a 10-year-old and adjust your replies on the feedback and questions you get in response.

'Parents' expectations or concerns might be completely different to the task you have been set and it is up to you to confirm what is being expected. I will give a small anecdote. Few years ago I went to see a mother who had delivered a baby about 12 hours ago. The baby had been vomiting and was diagnosed to have duodenal atresia. He also had a capillary haemangioma on his forehead. During my discussion, I realised the mother was more concerned about the haemangioma on the face then the duodenal atresia for which the baby needed urgent surgery. She felt that the duodenal atresia will be sorted and hence was not really a problem. It was an eye opener for me about difference in perspectives.

After initial introductions, I would start by finding a quiet place and check if that is suitable for both. I then continue with checking what the person knows already. "Can you please tell me what you have been told so far?" "How is X doing? How can I help?" This clarifies the agenda. I acknowledge their information and build on it. I would first describe a NORMAL situation of the problem to be discussed. I use simple drawing to explain concepts or anatomy of the topic under discussion (4 chambers of the heart with basic conduction pathway if arrhythmia is to be discussed). I use scenarios that are familiar from day-to-day life, that the other person may have experienced drawing similarities. Once the person is comfortable with that, I move to the abnormality, explaining it in brief simple terms, frequently checking I am being understood. I would ask them to repeat what they have understood. This works very well on most occasions.

It is usually good practice to give a very brief description of what is normal when describing a condition. This then allows you to explain how things or findings are different and their possible implications.

If the other person/role player is 'upset or angry', the **trick is not to interrupt them when they are venting their feelings**. Give them time and usually they will finish in less than a minute (it may seem like a lot more but bite your tongue and keep quiet, **continue attentive listening**) during this time you should have listened to and identified what is most important to them. You can then start by offering an apology, clearing the misunderstanding and finally moving on to the task you have been set.

Mention you would document the discussion in the notes – in law – if it is not documented—it is *not* done.

Breaking Bad News

It is a common scenario and one that you must be prepared for well. It can come in a number of ways and a generic overview will help you prepare for most situations.

What is bad news? It can mean different things to different people. 'Any information, which adversely and seriously affects an individual or if a message is given which reduces the options in an individual's future' is bad news. It can be a child has cancer, needs major surgery, may have brain damage, has chromosomal defect, etc. they all have serious life changing effects.

Patients/parents increasingly want as much information as possible regarding the diagnosis, treatment and side effects. They want the doctor to be honest, compassionate, caring, informative and HOPEFULL. They would like the information given in private setting with a supportive person present and with time for discussion if they want.

The normal response to bad news is Grief reaction in most individuals. During which the individual will go through the following emotions:

- Numbness and denial
- Anger
- Sadness
- Acceptance
- Hope

Do not open your consultation with: "I am sorry – I have some bad news" as I have often heard. Also leave on a positive note and there is always something positive in every situation.

You should be prepared to deal with each and respond appropriately. In the numbness and denial phase the person can go very quiet, "It cannot be true!", "Are you sure?" "Can there be a mistake?" You need to be quiet too and allow silence for the information to sink in and do not necessarily try and respond to each of the statements.

After appropriate pause, you can ask if they have heard of the condition and what they know about it? Explain in appropriate terms.

Anger is *not* directed at you in person but is unwittingly directed at the 'bearer' of news. Remain calm and reassure.

Hope is the most important feeling a person looks for at such. You do not have to give the last know complication or side effect of the illness or treatment but do *not* give false information. You will be marked down—in such a situation — admit your ignorance, arrange to come back after checking further information.

Do not give too much information – even if you think you have to tell them all, keep your eye contact and act on visual and verbal cues. Tell them as much as they want to know—keep in mind real life scenarios where there will be opportunities in the future to build on what has been said. In the examination same principles apply when you arrange to meet them again.

Always check the identity of the person you are speaking to and check the relationship to the child under discussion. Do *not* get this wrong as besides creating a lot of anxiety, you will be breaching patient confidentiality.

When given bad news – parents will always assume the worst, impending doom and gloom. Your task is to allow them to keep the situation in perspective and provide reassurance and hope.

There are no absolutes rights or wrongs to dealing with a communication scenario but some approaches are better accepted than others.

I will give you how I would do it. The scene is that you are the registrar on call in a District General Hospital (DGH). It is after 5 PM, your local haematologist rings to inform you that John, a 5-year-old boy who was admitted earlier in the day with bruising and lymphadenopathy, has been confirmed as suffering from acute lymphatic leukaemia (ALL). You have discussed this with your consultant and are now going to speak to John's parents.

Think for a few minutes and write down the main things you will do and say before reading on.

The set up in UK is that 'uncommon' conditions, i.e. malignancy, cardiac surgery, etc. are treated in fewer specialised hospital so as to increase the expertise available and get better results. These hospitals can be consulted, 24/7, as and when the need arises, joint care is planned and executed over the next few days, weeks and months. Patients are generally transferred to the specialised hospital at the earliest convenient time.

I suggest **before** you speak to the parents you contact the local oncology centre. Discuss with them John's illness and have a plan as to what will be done next so that you can explain to the parents. Request a senior nurse to accompany you during your conversation and remember to document in the notes afterwards what was discussed. Find a quiet room. Ask if they would like anyone else to be present. Once you break the news of 'ALL', parents will 'shut down' and will only be interested in 'Will John die *and* What will be done next?' If you do not know or cannot find an answer to any of their questions, i.e. prognosis and cure rates, be prepared to say you do not know but acknowledge that the information will be available to them when they see the 'specialist' at the other hospital.

Once prepared, invite the parents into a side room, where it will be quiet and arrange for not to be disturbed, hand over your bleep to a colleague.

I would open the discussion with introductions and ask them "How is John and what have they been told?" Check their understanding of the illness so far.

"We did some tests because of his bruising and I have the results of the test we did in the morning. The results are suggestive of a condition called Leukemia"... Pause.

I will keep quiet for 5–10 seconds after that and wait for their response. The parents may have heard of leukemia before and ask if it is 'cancer' or they may not know. If they do not I would carry on and say it is a type of cancer. Once the penny drops, parents are, understandably, very emotional. You need to keep quiet till they acknowledge that they are ready for further information. You should then explain what is to be done next. "Children, who have illness as John has, are treated at specialist hospitals. I have spoken with my counterpart there and have made an appointment for him to be seen there tomorrow". You will make arrangement for transport. For now you will carry on with treatment they have recommended. You should answer their other questions to the best of your ability but acknowledge your lack of knowledge where applicable.

The above model can be easily adapted for child with serious congenital cardiac defect requiring urgent surgery or a neonate requiring intensive care with 'cooling' for birth asphyxia available only at a few units.

Practice this and find out the arrangements in your local set up so you may be able to describe local practice. Moving on ....

We also communicate with our bodies—the body language. When conveying emotions, if our body language, tone of voice and words are not in synchrony, then the body language and tone of voice will be believed more than the spoken word. "Nice to meet you" said while looking away and mumbling with a limp hand shake and no eye contact—will be taken as 'insincere and not reliable'.

It is worth remembering that some accepted ways of mannerism may have different interpretation in different cultures.

Eye contact with our seniors eyes/gazing is considered rude and disrespectful in certain cultures, i.e. Indian. However, avoiding eye contact in the Western culture and specially during the exams can be misinterpreted as lack of confidence. Hence it is important to make good eye contact with the person you are speaking to. If you find looking into the eyes of another person uncomfortable, then you can fix your gaze at the persons shoulder or at their ears. This from a distance of more than a few feet will give the impression that you have eye contact and you will not suffer the penalty of being thought of as lacking confidence.

Empathy: You will see this mentioned repeatedly. It is difficult to know what it means and how to 'show' it. A definition I like is "The ability to put oneself into the mental shoes of another person to understand her emotions and feelings." For example, if you had to discuss and give results of a test, i.e. chromosomes, to a patient, think how you had felt in a similar situation may be when getting the marks for your last exam – the butterflies in the stomach, dry mouth, racing pulse, wondering what you are going to be told and how that might affect the future. During the communication scenarios put yourself in the other person's shoes and act how you would like to be spoken *with* and *not* to yourself.

Therefore in a successful communication exercise you will:
- **Familiarize yourself with the background**
- **Have some knowledge of management options**
- **Introduce yourself**
- **Check how the 'person' would like to be addressed**
- **Make eye contact**
- **Confirm the identity of the person and cross check relationship with the child**
- **Confirm the task set, negotiate if else is required**
- **Explain in small byte sized bits of information** (30 seconds bytes)
- **Use pause and silence to emphasize information**

- **Regularly checking the message is being understood**
- **Look out for verbal and nonverbal cue**
- **Ask for repeating what they have understood**
- **Offer to provide information in form of leaflets**
- **Finish and have an appropriate summarizing at end**
- **Be sensitive and do not interrupt**
- **Try and remain positive**
- **Make a safety net—arrange to review if required.**

Remember the exam situation is very artificial. To an extent it is a 'play/ drama', with each member having a designated role. You, the examiner, patient or role player. The latter two work/act to a script with some free play allowed. You have to do the same.

This will improve with practice.

Guru Mantra

- Make eye contact—be aware of your body language
- Clarify and check 'patient/role player' understanding of the topic
- Do not speak for more than 30 seconds before checking comprehension.

Communication Scenarios

The following scenarios are for role playing with colleagues. If you can video them – reviewing them will be even more helpful.

Useful images are provided throughout the book. Images and photographs are not provided in the communication station in the clinical examination but these will be useful in video station and even the MRCPCH written examination.

The information in the following chapters is confidential and privileged. You are expected to follow your Medical Council guidelines on Patient confidentiality. By continuing you accept your responsibility.

Each case is divided into four parts.

Work through each with one or two colleague acting different parts and feeding back. Just reading them through will not be as useful.

Use a recording device (can be your mobile) to check what you sound like when speaking. It will be an 'eye' opener.

CHILD PROTECTION / WITHHOLDING TREATMENT

Information given to the candidate

You are the paediatric registrar working in a District General Hospital. You are working in the outpatient clinic today. You are about to speak to Ms Sandra James, who has come to see you without Cody, her son. Cody is 6-year-old and is known to have congenital hypothyroidism. He is on 75 mcg of oral thyroxine once a day.

Results of blood investigations done 4 days ago show: TSH >100 mIU/L. High TSH results were also noted on earlier occasions.

Please discuss the implications of this result with Cody's mother

You are not expected to gather any more history but may answer any queries that the mother may raise.

You have 9 minutes to complete the station; a warning bell will be given at 7 minutes (SP).

Information available to the mother (actress)

You are the mother with 3 young children and are divorced. Minimal support is available and you find it hard to work and manage the family. You feel that Cody is well and it is not good to give medicines to a child regularly. They may get used to the medicine and then may need more of it in the future.

You were explained about the diagnosis but did not understand the details of the explanation as to why long term medication will be necessary for Cody. When informed about the results you raise a query whether the result is erroneous.

You are worried that the medical team may feel that you are an incompetent mother and social services will 'take away' your child. You need to be reassured by the candidate that social services can also give support and can contribute by providing additional support.

You are expected to exhibit controlled emotions but you need not volunteer any other information unless specifically asked.

What is expected from the candidate?

• Introduces self to the mother and asks about the well-being of the child. Can take a lead from how she replies as how to address her.
• Refers to the actress/role player—as Ms James or Sandra and not as mum or mother.
• Addresses the child by his name 'Cody'· Explains and AGREE the agenda for the clinic discussion

- Mentions about the result and its implications
- Checks mother's understanding about Cody's diagnosis and need for regular medications
- Check why she *may* not be giving Cody the required dose.
- Gives a clear management plan and follow-up plans, preferable offer to write down the frequency and dosage.
- Acknowledge that laboratory results can be erroneous at times but high TSH has been noted earlier as well. *Do not* sound as if accusing.
- Does not gather further history or unnecessary information
- Does not give false reassurance that social service involvement is not necessary
- Summarises the discussion and addresses any concern raised by the mother *frequently checks mother's understanding*.
- *Avoids monologue*—speak not for more than 30 seconds before checking understanding or seeking any questions.
- Does not use medical jargon.

GENERAL NOTE

If you are not familiar with the set up in UK, a few details about Child support/ surveillance/protection.

At birth all children have a newborn screening physical examination and on day 5 a heel prick blood test, Guthrie's test is done for Hypothyroidism, Cystic Fibrosis, Phenylketonuria, MCAD and Sickle cell disease in certain areas. A child's growth and development is supported and monitored by Health Visitors and General Practitioners.

Social services, via social workers, provide financial and other support to families in need. Social services also have the authority to institute procedures where children may be highlighted and given extra help as 'Children in Need' or be removed from a family and put in '**Care**', i.e. under Government responsibility for a period of time or permanently, if the circumstances so demand. This can be if the child in not being cared for appropriately, is neglected, abused physically or emotionally, is not given prescribed medications. Hence parents generally are vary of social services/workers and do not like them (*see* appendix)

A suggested approach to this station (in details)

C: Candidate

S: Sandra or Ms James

C: Good morning, I am Dr XXX, one of the paediatric registrars working in the hospital. Thanks for coming today, how would you like to be addressed?

S: Thanks doctor, please call me Sandra. I am bit worried about this urgent clinic appointment today.

C: Hello Sandra. There is no need to be worried. How are you and did you have to make lot of changes to come at short notice?

S: I am a bit stressed and yes I had to leave my other two children with my mother.

C: How is Cody?

S: Oh! Cody is well and has gone to school.

C: Thanks and good to know that Cody is ok. I want to discuss the results of the blood tests he had a few days ago. In the test we measure how much medicine he is getting by a test called 'TSH'. The results of 'TSH' suggest that Cody is not getting enough medicine to keep his hormone level normal.

S: You are right doctor; I do forget to give Cody the tablets every day and it is really difficult to remember, I have 3 small children you see. Are you sure the results are correct? I know of other friends whose test results have been wrong.

Little pause.

C: Sandra, this is possible. However, the laboratory does check all results that are abnormal before sending them to doctors. Cody also had high results on tests done before. Also as you mentioned that Cody does not get his medicine daily so his hormone level are likely to be low and the test result abnormal.

S: I do *not* like giving medicine to Cody, my little child daily. I feel he is well at present, why unnecessarily give medicine?

C: Sandra how much do you remember about Cody's illness/diagnosis?

S: Not a lot, I know Cody was lacking some hormone in his body but he must better by now. Is not he? Can you tell me again what is wrong with Cody?

C: Sandra, It is common to get confused about details of what we are told over a period. Cody has got a condition called "congenital hypothyroidism". That means from the time of his birth Cody cannot produce a hormone called Thyroxine. Thyroxine is very important for the proper growth and development of a person and Cody will need to take the medicine all his life. That is the medicine he has to take every day. This hormone helps in his growth, development of the brain and helps in learning.

S: I feel like a very bad mother now that Cody's brain is damaged because of me.

C: Sandra please do not feel that way, I am sure you are a good mother and try your best to make sure your children are healthy. Is there any other way we can help you to make sure Cody gets his medicine.

S: Are you going to inform the social services about my family, I really do not like their involvement as they will take Cody away from me. (Sobs)

(Pause, you may offer a tissue)

C: Sandra I am sorry you feel that way about the social services. They can actually be a very helpful resource by providing some extra child care help and financial support so as to help the situation. However, I will respect your views and do not feel Social service involvement is necessary as yet *but* **I will discuss this with my Consultant Mr Thompson.** However, discussing with Social services may be necessary at a later stage.

S: Ok

C: How do you feel about some extra support from the community nursing team in monitoring that Cody is taking the medicines and also that a regular supply of medicine is available from the local doctor.

S: (Reluctantly) Yes, that would be helpful. So, what happens now?

C: Do *not* use the medicine you have at home. I will confirm the right dose for Cody and give you a fresh prescription for some ready supply of thyroxine. We also need to organise further blood tests in a few weeks and a date for follow-up in this clinic. I will also mention about this discussion to Dr Thomson, Cody's consultant.
(The 7 minutes alarm is sounded and you summarise the discussion)

S: Doctor is Cody going to be fine?

C: Sandra he should remain well given the right treatment. We will need to monitor Cody's progress closely, make sure that he remains well, his educational achievements are good and will be **only able to do it with your help**.

S: Thanks doctor.

C: Sandra just to summarise what we discussed today; Cody will need life-long thyroxine to maintain good health. We will fix a date for the repeat blood tests and then a follow-up date. The community nursing team will provide some support to help you manage Cody's medical condition. Is there anything I can help with you today.

S: No doctor, thank you.

C: Thanks Sandra, please feel free to get back to me through Dr Thompson's secretary and I will arrange for some leaflets about Hypothyroidism for you before you leave the clinic today. Thank you.

NOTE

Practice this but use your own language and phrases that you feel comfortable with. Print out the sheet and work in groups of three if possible. Two doing the role play and the third person observing and able to give feedback on:

- *How it felt 'watching' the interaction*
- *Commenting on the speech*
- *Body language*
- *Timing.*

All three do not have to be doctors.

NONACCIDENTAL INJURY (NAI)

Information given to the candidate

Two and a half year old girl Shannon brought to the hospital A&E by grandmother with multiple bruises of different size and colour on trunk and back. Child admitted as suspected of nonaccidental injury late previous night. Further investigations have not been organized yet. Mother does not know of child being admitted for NAI and has come to collect the child. She thinks the girl has had a viral rash and child was seen in hospital to rule out 'meningitis' as seen on TV.

You have been asked to see Shannon's mother who has just arrived. Shannon was brought to the hospital by her grandmother and admitted late previous night with multiple bruises of different size and colour, highly suspicious of non accidental injury.

Your task is to explain to mother your suspicion and your management plan

You are not expected to gather any more history but may answer any queries that Shannon's mother may raise during the discussion.

You have 9 minutes to complete the station; a warning bell will be given at 7 minutes(AG).

Information available to mother (actor)

You are Josephine, 21-year-old, mother of Shannon, living with a new boy friend for past 6 months. You allow your ex-partner's mother to have contact with Shannon, her grand-daughter, and allow Shannon to spend the odd night at her home.

Shannon was with her grandmother the day before as you had to go to a party. You got a call saying Shannon was being taken to hospital to be checked out as she had developed a bruise.

- Say you are in a hurry and would like to leave ASAP as you have to get 'somewhere'.
- Ask what do they mean by NAI?
- Are they accusing you of hurting your child?
- You will take them to court and are going to walk out with the child.
- After some discussion you reluctantly agree to keep Shannon in hospital
- You mention you have been stressed and have hit Shannon at times.
- You have also noted change in Shannon's behavior, she is clingy, tearful.
- Your current boy friend has a short temper and you have had arguments with him.

What is expected from the candidate?
Examiners/Observers
- Appropriate greeting
- Arranges for a quiet room, not disturbed by bleep.
- Requests a nurse or sister looking after child to accompany.
- Adequate explanation of bruises and further plan of NAI:
  - Discuss with seniors
  - Social service
  - Skeletal survey
  - Clotting studies
  - Not accusing mother of injury
- Does not allow child to be removed from hospital.
- Sympathetic and seeks other information about feeling of mother
- Information about partner
- Summarizes at the end

GENERAL NOTE

Typical bruises seen in children with suspected Nonaccidental Injury. Bruising on the pinna of external ear is highly suspicious of nonaccidental nature (*see* body map in Appendix).

You will not have photographs in the communication station but may get similar images in your video station or in your written part II.

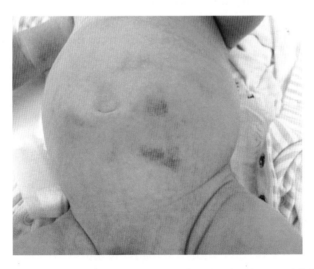

Fig. 4: A 4-month-old baby with bruising on abdomen. Bruising in a 'non-mobile' infant is generally serious and needs appropriate follow through

PYLORIC STENOSIS

Scene

Information given to the candidate

Henry, 5-week-old, male infant admitted with 2 week history of projectile vomiting. He was moderately dehydrated. Peristaltic waves noted in epigastric region. Test feed is 'positive'. Blood chemistry: pH: 7.45, pO_2: 6 kPa, pCO_2: 7 kPa, HCO_3: 41 mEq/L, BXs: 28. Na: 145, Cl: 90, K: 3.3, Ur: 7 (all in mmol/L), Cr: 35 μmol/L. A diagnosis of pyloric stenosis has been made.

Father has refused the SHO, to go to the 'nearest' surgical unit in a nearby hospital, (Teaching Hospital).

You are the registrar on duty working in a medium size DGH. You have come to see father of Henry to tell him of the diagnosis and to transfer him to paediatric surgical unit at nearby large teaching hospital for surgery. The other paediatric surgical unit is 150 miles away.

Your task is to explain to father the diagnosis and the need for surgery at nearby paediatric surgical hospital, part of a large teaching hospital set up.

You are not expected to gather any more history but may answer any queries that Henry's father may raise during the discussion.

You have 9 minutes to complete the station; a warning bell will be given at 7 minutes (AG).

Information available to father (actor)

You are father of Henry, who has been admitted with vomiting. You are very worried and feel Henry is very unwell and may die as he is so unwell. You have seen 5 doctors in last two weeks and they all said he had a 'tummy bug'.

Two years ago your sister and her new born baby died during at birth at a nearby teaching hospital. You feel the hospital was very careless and 'killed' your sister and niece. You do not want to go there again.

- You want to know how ill Henry is and is he going to die.
- What do all the results mean and what is being done.
- Why did doctors before did not pick it up?
- What is the next step? When will the surgery be? Why is being delayed? Where will it be? You do not want to go to the 'teaching hospital'.
- Explain why you do not want to go – **if the doctors asks you for your reasons**. Do not come out with it spontaneously.
- If the reason is asked and handled sensitively and with adequate explanation – you MAY agree to go to the 'teaching hospital'.
- Negotiate you would like to come back as soon after surgery as possible.

What is expected from the candidate?

Examiners/Observers

Look for
- Non jargonistic explanation of pyloric stenosis.
- Adequate explanation of blood chemistry
- Delay in surgery due to stabilisation of 'chemistry'.
- Checks for understanding.
- Accepts patient autonomy of not wanting to go to a a particular hospital
- Exploring of refusal to go to surgical unit.
- Negotiation of care plan with father – joint care.
- Summarizing at end.

PERINATAL ASPHYXIA

Information given to the candidate

Mary, a 23-year-old primigravida, had prolonged labour. She gave birth to a term baby by an emergency caesarean section under spinal regional anaesthesia, following an attempted ventouse delivery. The baby was covered in meconium and required resuscitation with positive pressure ventilation and cardiac massage. First gasp at 10 minutes. Cord pH: 6.91. Decision has been taken to transfer him to regional neonatal unit for cooling.

You are in the delivery suite and have resuscitated a male infant with severe birth asphyxia. Gasp at 10 minutes. Cord pH: 6.91.

You have to speak to baby's parents to explain what has happened and ask for permission for transfer and cooling.

You are not expected to gather any more history but may answer any queries that Henry's father may raise during the discussion.

You have 9 minutes to complete the station; a warning bell will be given at 7 minutes (NM).

Information available to mother (actor)

You are Mary, 23-year-old, you have just birth to a baby boy. There was 'difficulty' during the last hour of delivery. Your baby has not cried and doctors have been 'treating' him. They have been whispering and you are very concerned. You partner is with you.

You are both teachers.
You want to know:
• Why is he not crying
• Is he dead? Is he going to be alright?
• Why does he need to be transferred?
• What is cooling?
• Can your partner go with the baby?
• What will happen in future? Will he be mentally retarded?

What is expected from the candidate?
Examiners/Observers
Look for:

• Nonjargonistic explanation of birth asphyxia
• Adequate explanation of blood chemistry
• Explains Cooling—Hypothermia as treatment for asphyxia
• Checks for understanding.
• Empathic
• Summarizing at end

GENERAL NOTE

In therapeutic cooling or 'hypothermia' the infant is cooled to between 33°C and 35°C, with the aim of preventing further neuronal loss in the days following the hypoxic injury.

Whole body is cooled with a blanket or mattress (or sometimes by cooling the head only with a purpose made cap). Core temperature is continuously monitored using a rectal or nasopharyngeal thermometer.

Treatment is started as soon as possible after diagnosis, usually within 6 hours of birth, and continued for approximately 72 hours. The infant is then slowly warmed to normal body temperature.

The facility for cooling is not available in all units where babies are delivered. In infants subjected to perinatal asphyxia and meeting criterion for cooling transfer is arranged. Prior to transfer to the specialist unit for 'active' cooling, the infants are commenced on 'passive cooling' during which external heating is turned off and the temperature of the baby monitored carefully. Definite benefits have been reported in neurological outcomes with increase of survival without neurological abnormality increasing from 28 to 44%. There was lower rates of cerebral palsy in infants treated by cooling.

References

http://www.mrc.ac.uk/About/AnnualReview09-10/SevenAges/Baby/Cooling/index.htm

https://www.npeu.ox.ac.uk/files/downloads/tobyregister/TOBY-Register-Cooling-PIL.pdf

http://www.nice.org.uk/guidance/index.jsp?action=article&o=47222

ANGRY PARENTS—RESPIRATORY ARREST

Information given to the candidate

Stewart, one month old baby is admitted to ward as parents are concerned about his feeding.

You are ST3 who has looked after Stewart. He is a 1 month baby with aortic stenosis, mild hyoplasia of the aortic arch. He underwent aortic valvolpasty at the regional cardiac centre 3 weeks ago. He was admitted earlier with evidence of congestive cardiac failure. During insertion of nasogastric tube by a nurse, he had a respiratory arrest plus minimal bleeding from his nostril. You have resuscitated him and Stewart is now stable. You feel you have done a good job and have saved his life.

You have to explain to father what has happened, as he was present when Stewart stopped breathing as nasogastric tube was being inserted and has been watching from outside the cubicle.

You are not expected to gather any more history but may answer any queries that Stewart's father may raise during the discussion.

You have 9 minutes to complete the station; a warning bell will be given at 7 minutes (NM).

Information available to father (actor)

You are John, father of Stewart. You brought your son into hospital as he was not feeding well. You are worried as he was unwell a few days after birth and was brought to the same hospital. You feel nobody could identify the illness for 2 days till Stewart deteriorated when he was transferred to another 'specialist' hospital. You were told there that he has narrowing of one of his heart valves and he underwent an emergency operation. He was given medicines to take. He was well till about 2 days ago when he developed difficulty in breathing and feeding. The doctors explained about few things that are wrong now and need treating.

- You are not sure but feel you have to agree.
- You notice the nurse pass a tube into the nose. Stewart cries and arches his back. He then stops crying and his colour turns blue. Nurse presses an alarm button.
- Lots of other people arrive, you are ignored as they 'work' with the baby. It seems like a 'lifetime' for the baby to become pink, you have not heard him cry.
- You are very worried and angry. Has the episode affected him in any way and made his condition worse.

- You feel this hospital is 'Not good' and is not capable of looking after your child.
- You want your child transferred to the 'specialist' hospital as last time
- If that is not possible you want him to go to another hospital where the staff are better and 'know' what they are doing.
- You have lost all confidence in the staff of this hospital
- You want to know 'why was there blood' from the baby's nose before he stopped breathing. Who was responsible and what will be done about that.
- **You initially want to be transferred as soon as possible *but* will later agree to stay if the doctor offers to accept your request but then manages to convince you that the episode was unexpected but a known side effect of nasogastric tube insertion, further management and transfer, if needed, is agreed.**
- **You thank the doctor in the end and apologize for your outburst.**

What is expected from the candidate?
Examiners/Observers

- Appropriate greeting, check's identity
- Shows Stewart and explains he is stable now.
- Arranges for a quiet room, not disturbed by bleep.
- Requests a nurse or sister looking after baby to accompany.
- Gives father opportunity to have his say and desire to be transferred
- Does not interrupt or retaliate with corrections
- Listens sympathetically
- Apologizes to father
- Emphasizes baby is stable now and gives details of respiratory arrest
- Admits possible error in technique of NG insertion – will look into it
- This may have competency issues will also discuss with consultant
- Explains will explore but the need, problems and difficulties in transferring to specialist unit
- Confirms management plan with father
- Summarizes discussion and agreement
- Arranges to review baby later
- Mention will documents in the notes

GENERAL NOTE
Comments on the case
This is a difficult scenario. Here the father's perception is that the hospital cannot provide adequate care as the baby had to be transferred to a specialist hospital for 'proper treatment'.

- This has to be put in perspective.
- Remain quiet during angry outburst.
- The error has to be acknowledged.
- Apology for the mistake.
- Put the need for specialist hospital in context and not to agree to transfer to tertiary hospital. You may agree to offer another hospital as part of discussion and negotiation.

GOOD MEDICAL PRACTICE—MEDICAL RECORDS

Information given to the candidate

You are the paediatric ST4 working in a District General Hospital. You are to talk to Dr John Garlick, a FY2 (junior colleague) working in the department. John has been noted to make changes in the medical notes of a few children. A recent incident was picked up by a ward nurse when he changed blood pressure recording in the notes 2 days later. You have spoken to other registrars who have voiced a similar concern. It has also been noted that John has been absent from work and late to come to work on 7 occasions in the last month.

Please speak to John, explain the implications of changing medical notes and put some strategies in place to prevent recurrence of this.

You are not expected to gather any more history but may answer any queries that John may raise during the discussion.

You have 9 minutes to complete the station; a warning bell will be given at 7 minutes (SP).

Information available to the FY2 doctor (actor)

You are Dr John Garlick, a FY2 trainee in paediatrics. You try to work hard but feels working with children is quite challenging. You felt that everything needs to be recorded in medical notes and therefore made retrospective additions in the medical notes. You feel that you are well supported by the senior colleagues.

When explained that medical notes are a legal document you become concerned and are scared. You request the ST4 colleague not to inform the consultant as you feel you may lose your job.

You want to know what happens from here and will expect to hear about GMC good medical practice code but do not ask about it.

You are expected to exhibit controlled emotions. You are not expected to give any personal information about your social life. You have recently broken up with your girlfriend and had a very stressful time and found it hard to attend work but you choose not to bring it up during the discussion.

What is expected from the candidate?

- Introduces self and clearly mentions aim for the discussion
- Exhibits empathy towards a struggling colleague and enquires about his well being but does not probe into John's social/personal life.
- Appreciates John's contribution to the team
- Clearly asks John whether he made alterations in notes

- Mentions that medical notes are a legal document and should not be altered and entries made later should be clearly dated and signed
- Reassures about support to be provided
- Do not give false reassurance that the consultant will not be informed as requested
- Mentions this is a learning opportunity for John
- Clear plan for improvement
- Mentions GMC good medical practice
- Summarises the discussion and offers to update John about his progress
- Does not use medical jargon – *but* should use adequate medical terminology as is *speaking* to a *doctor*. Too much lay talk can be counterproductive.

GENERAL NOTE

General Medical Council (GMC) is the regulatory body for medical profession in UK. Details of advice from GMC can be found on www.gmc-uk.org

INTRODUCTION OF A NEW DRUG THERAPY IN A PATIENT WITH DIABETES

Information given to the candidate

You are the paediatric ST4 working in a District General Hospital. You are working in the outpatient clinic today. You are about to speak to Miss Chloe Bolton, a 15-year-old girl with Type1 diabetes mellitus on insulin. As part of her yearly review, urine test was done which revealed microalbuminuria. Her latest HbA1C is 8.6 mmol/L. It was decided that Chloe would benefit from regular Lisinopril therapy (ACE inhibitor).

Chloe has been invited for a clinic appointment.

You need to discuss with Chloe about her urine results and the need for adding Lisinopril therapy

You are not expected to gather any more history but may answer any queries that the Chloe may raise during the discussion.

You have 9 minutes to complete the station; a warning bell will be given at 7 minutes (SP).

Information available to Miss Chloe Bolton (Actress/Patient)

You are Miss Chloe Bolton, 15-year-old girl with Type1 diabetes mellitus on twice daily insulin therapy. You have been a diabetic for 10 years, generally have good control of your diabetes and have good support from your parents. You are a bit worried why you have been called back to the clinic suddenly.

You have good understanding of diabetes but do not know anything about this microalbuminuria and expect a simple explanation about this from the doctor.

When the doctor informs about the need for introduction of a new medicine you want to know why this is needed as your diabetes is under control. You will also want to know what problems may arise with this medicine.

You are not sure that this is necessary and wants to discuss with your parents. You want an opportunity to come back and meet the doctor after a week with your decision.

You are expected to exhibit controlled emotions but is not supposed to volunteer any other information unless specifically asked.

What is expected from the candidate?

- Introduces self to Chloe and thanks her for coming to the clinic at short notice.
- Explains the agenda for the clinic discussion, viz. what does micro-albuminuria mean and why it is important for Chloe's diabetes?
- Mentions about the result and its implications

- Checks Chloe's understanding about the results and offers a simple explanation about the protein in urine.
- Informs about the need for Lisinopril for protection from further effects of diabetic nephropathy.
- While acknowledge that Lisinopril is important but gives enough scope to Chloe to clarify her concerns and offers opportunity to come back at a later date with her decision.
- Does not make up side effects (if not known) but offers to consult a book and inform Chloe by letter or during the next discussion session.
- Does not gather further history or unnecessary information
- Does not push for the medicine to be started at that time but shows empathy and understanding needed to deal with children with a chronic condition.
- Summarises the discussion and addresses any concern raised by Chloe
- Agrees to meet up with Chloe at a specified date to start the medicine.
- *Avoids monologue* – **speak not for more than 30 seconds before checking understanding or seeking any questions.**
- Does not use medical jargon

GENERAL NOTE

Foundation doctors (FY1 and FY2) are immediately after completing the MBBS and last 2 years.

It is important to follow the general communication guidelines.

CHILD SAFETY/TELEPHONIC CONVERSATION WITH A PARENT

Information given to the candidate

You are the paediatric registrar working in a District General Hospital. You are on call at night. You have been busy with a neonatal resuscitation. Your SHO informs you she has seen a 23-day-old baby called Alfie in the Emergency department earlier. Alfie had rolled off himself from a changing mattress and suffered mild head injury. She was happy with Alfie's clinical condition but requests you to see the baby as she is not comfortable with such a young infant.

You reach the Emergency department 40 minutes later and are informed by the nurse that Alfie has been gone, taken home by his father Mr Onions against medical advice. The observations recoded in the notes were within normal limits.

You, the candidate, need to call Mr Onions over the phone explaining that Alfie needs to brought back to the hospital for reassessment straight away.

You are not expected to gather any more history but may answer any queries that the father may raise. Please dial 7452 and wait for an answer.

You have 9 minutes to complete the station; a warning bell will be given at 7 minutes (SP).

Information available to the father (actor)

You are Mr Onions, father of Alfie. You wife has been unwell since birth of Alfie and you have a 2-year-old daughter. At 10 pm tonight you were changing Alfie's nappy on a changing mat. He slipped and fell about 2 feet from a table on to a thick carpeted floor. He cried straight away but was easily consoled, did not vomit and no swelling was noted. You felt remorseful and sought medical advice straight away, taking him to the local hospital. You do not drive and a kind neighbour brought two of you to the hospital.

A doctor examined Alfie and felt he was concerned that there was bruise on the forehead. The doctor requested you to wait as he wanted his senior colleague (i.e. the candidate) to have a look at Alfie. The doctor was also worried that Alfie has not fed since the time of the fall.

As Alfie remained well and had fed well you felt that there was no further medical intervention was needed. Your neighbour was getting late hence you came back home. Alfie is fine now and sleeping.

An apology is expected from the candidate at the outset explaining the circumstances for the unavoidable delay. The candidate may reiterate the history to check he has got the facts right. You do not want to go back to the hospital as there is no available transport and you do not have enough money to call a taxi. You are further worried about the child care arrangement for your other child as your wife is unwell.

The candidate needs to convince you that it is very important that Alfie is brought back to the hospital for the reassessment as signs and symptoms may be falsely reassuring in a baby with head injury.

You are expected to exhibit controlled emotions and anger but if convinced by the candidate that Alfie may come to harm and further steps may need to be initiated if non-compliant with the request, you will reluctantly agree to come back.

What is expected from the candidate?
- Introduces self to the Mr Onions over the phone and asks about the well-being of the child.
- Refers the actor as Mr Onions and not as dad or father.
- Addresses the child by his name 'Alfie'
- Explains the agenda for the telephone discussion
- Offers a clear apology for the delay due to unavoidable circumstances.
- Mentions about the need for the reassessment and hence need for Alfie to be brought back to the hospital
- Checks Mr Onions' understanding about Alfie's head injury and need for the senior review.
- Express empathy and an understanding of the difficult situation Mr Onions is in
- Does not agree that Alfie is well at home and therefore there is no need for reassessment thus do not compromise Alfie's health
- May offer an alternative that Mr Onions may be able to claim back the fare for the taxi from the hospital but will need to confirm it with the hospital manager (usually a senior nurse)
- May also want to involve the on-call consultant if faced with a difficult parent for advice and support.
- May explain the need to involve police or social services if Mr Onions remains non-compliant after a proper explanation
- Summarises the discussion and addresses any concern raised by the father
- Does not use medical jargon

GENERAL NOTE
A 23-day-old baby cannot roll over and any such vague history should set the alarm bells ringing about potential child abuse concerns.
- *A 4-week-old baby "rolled over" and fell out of bed.*
- *A 4-month-old crawled and reached the hot cup of tea and was scalded*

It is important to know the development milestones so as to be able to judge if the suggested mode of injury is feasible for a child of particular age.

Developmental key stages	
• Fixing and smiling	6 weeks
• Rolling over	5 months
• Reaching out	5 months
• Transferring	6 months
• Sitting	7 months
• Crawling	8–9 months
• Walking with support	1 year

INTRODUCTION OF A NEW DRUG THERAPY IN A PATIENT WITH NEPHROTIC SYNDROME— POOR COMPLIANCE

Information given to the candidate

You are the paediatric ST4 working in a District General Hospital. You are working in the outpatient clinic today. You are about to speak to Miss Chloe Charlton, a 15-year-old girl with Nephrotic syndrome, due to minimal change on histology, on oral steroids. She has relapsed for the third time and the decision is to start her on Levamisole.

Chloe has been invited for a clinic appointment.

You need to discuss with Chloe about her urine results and the need for changing Levamisole therapy

You are not expected to gather any more history but may answer any queries that the Chloe may raise during the discussion.

You have 9 minutes to complete the station; a warning bell will be given at 7 minutes (AG).

Information available to Miss Chloe Charlton (actress/patient)

You are Miss Chloe Charlton, 15 years old girl with nephrotic syndrome. You are a bit worried why you have been called back to the clinic suddenly.

You were diagnosed about 8 years ago. You responded to medication, oral steroids, and were well till 6 months ago. You then felt unwell and were told that the Nephrotic syndrome had relapsed. You were given Steroid tablets again which you took for only 3 weeks instead of three months. You stopped as you felt better and they made you gain weight. You again relapsed and stopped the steroids again after 3 weeks.

You have some understanding of nephrotic syndrome but do not know anything about the need to taking steroid medicine for 3 months when you get better in 2 weeks.

You have *not* told the doctors so far that you are *not* taking the steroid tablets as you were advised.

You are worried about getting fat and being teased at school. The tablets also make you agitated and cause you to have arguments with your parents and friends.

You will be willing to take the medications if someone explains 'properly' why they are important.

You will also want to know what problems may arise with this medicine. You are not sure that this is necessary and wants to discuss with your parents. You want an opportunity to come back and meet the doctor after a week with your decision.

You are expected to exhibit controlled emotions but is not supposed to volunteer any other information unless specifically asked.

What is expected from the candidate?

- Introduces self to Chloe and thanks Chloe for coming to the clinic at short notice.
- Explains the agenda for the clinic discussion, viz. what relapse of nephrotic syndrome is.
- Mentions about the result and its implications
- Checks Chloe understands about the results and offers a simple explanation about the protein in urine.
- Try and ascertain IF and *Why* she may *not* be complying with medication.
- Informs about the need for Levamisole for recurrent relapse.
- While acknowledge that introduction of Levamisole is important; but gives enough scope to Chloe to clarify her concerns and offers opportunity to come back at a later date with her decision.
- Does not make up side effects (if not known) but offers to consult a book and inform Chloe by letter or during the next discussion session.
- Does not gather further history or unnecessary information
- **Does not push for the medicine** to be started at that time but shows empathy and understanding needed to deal with children with a chronic condition.
- Summarises the discussion and addresses any concern raised by Chloe
- Agrees to meet up with Chloe at a specified date to start the medicine.
- *Avoids monologue* – **speak not for more than 30 seconds before checking understanding or seeking any questions.**
- Does not use medical jargon
- **Discussion regarding Levamisole may not be needed if finds that patient is not taking steroid**

GENERAL NOTE
Nephrotic syndrome

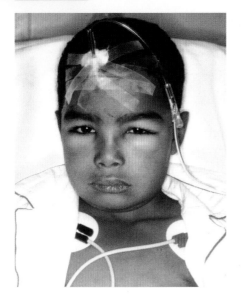

Fig. 5

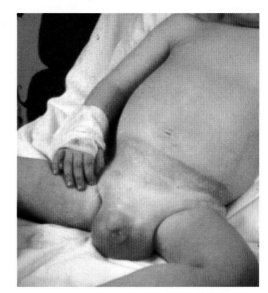

Fig. 6

To note
Puffy eye, scrotal oedema, abdominal wall oedema.

Management

- Medications – use of steroids. 2nd line immunosuppressive
- Nutrition
- Penicillin prophylaxis
- Pneumococcal vaccination
- Indications for biopsy

It is important to follow the general communication guidelines on communication.

EXPLAINING BENIGN ROLANDIC EPILEPSY

Information given to the candidate

You are the paediatric registrar working in the outpatient clinic today. You will be talking to mother of 5-year-old Millie who had presented with abnormal vocalisation with jerky movements noticed while she was asleep. She was admitted to paediatric ward and an EEG was arranged. The EEG shows centro-temporal spikes suggestive of Benign Rolandic epilepsy.

You will discuss the diagnosis with the mother Ms Grant who is anxious to know about the EEG results and what it means for Millie.

You are not expected to gather any further medical history but answer any queries that may arise during the discussion.

You have 9 minutes to complete the station; a warning bell will be given at 7 minutes (DR).

Information available to the mother (actor)

You are Ms Rebecca Grant, mother of Millie. Millie has been having abnormal episodes of making incomprehensible noises during her sleep along with some jerky movements. She was admitted to hospital and blood investigations were normal. Millie was discharged with a plan for outpatient EEG appointment. The EEG has been done and you are very anxious to find about the results. No one explained to you why the EEG was requested and about the results so far.

You expect an apology for *not* having being explained the management plan about Millie earlier. When explained that Millie has Benign Rolandic epilepsy, you become very scared as your friend's child has epilepsy and has learning disability and needs to wear a helmet all the time.

You need to be reassured that observation is all that will be necessary at present and Millie is likely to grow out of the condition. You want to know whether Millie can die in her sleep.

You will enquire about the need for lifestyle changes if the candidate does not bring it up during the discussion.

You are expected to exhibit controlled emotions. You are not expected to give any other personal information about yourself or Millie.

What is expected from the candidate?
- Introduces self to the mother and asks about the well-being of Millie.
- Can take a lead from how she replies as how to address her?
- Refers to the actress/role player – as Ms Grant or Rebecca and not as mum or mother.

- Addresses the child by her name 'Millie'
- Explains and AGREE the agenda for the clinic discussion
- Offers an apology that things were not explained properly earlier
- Mentions about the result of the EEG and its implications
- Checks mother understands about Millie's diagnosis and reassures mother that Millie's epilepsy is clearly different from her friend's child's epilepsy.
- **Checks if mother has any specific concerns or worries**
- Reassures that Millie will not die in her sleep, requires no medications and monitoring is all that is required at present
- Also explains that is likely to grow out of this and has a good prognosis.
- Gives a clear management plan and follow-up plans.
- Does not gather further history or unnecessary information
- Summarises the discussion and addresses any other concerns raised by the mother
- *Frequently checks mother's understanding.*
- *Avoids monologue*—speak not for more than 30 seconds before checking understanding or seeking any questions.
- Does not use medical jargon

AUDIT PROJECT DISCUSSION WITH F2/SHO

Information given to the candidate

You are the paediatric ST4 working in a District General Hospital. You are to speak to Dr Amit, F2/SHO working in the team. He would like to discuss an audit project he would like to do with you.

Task: Discuss with Dr Amit his project and advice him on the best course of action.

You are not expected to gather any more history but may answer any queries that may raise during the discussion.

You have 9 minutes to complete the station; a warning bell will be given at 7 minutes (AG).

Information available to Dr Amit

You wish to audit the effect of insulin infusion and metformin (oral hypoglycaemic agent) on children admitted to hospital over next 3 months.

You want to know:
- Why is yours not an audit project
- Difference between audit and research
- How do you organise an audit project
- Why do you need permission

If it is *not* mentioned:
- Ask

You need not volunteer any other information unless specifically asked.

What is expected from the candidate?
- Introduces self to role player.
- Explains the agenda/reason for meeting
- Clarify roles and identify topics to discuss
- Checks Amit's understanding of Audit and research and clarifies.
- Clarifies that the project as conceieved is a research project and *not* an audit.
- New information vs testing against 'gold' standard.
- Highlights difference between Type 1 and type 2 diabetes, role of oral anti-diabetic drugs in children.
- Unethical to give medication that we know are not effective
- Consent for involving patients.
- Does not make up information—but offers to consult and inform during the next discussion session.
- Agrees to meet again.

- Does not gather further history or unnecessary information
- Summarises the discussion and addresses any concern raised
- Agrees to arrange meeting for further information and advice to do literature search.
- *Avoids monologue* – **speak not for more than 30 seconds before checking understanding or seeking any questions.**
- Does not use medical jargon

GENERAL NOTE

Audit is central to clinical governance and in improving patient care.

AUDIT AND RESEARCH

Research: ' *a structured activity which is intended to provide new knowledge which is generalisable (i.e. of value to others in a similar situation) and intended for wider dissemination* ' (Department of Health, 2002)

Clinical audit: '*a quality improvement process that seeks to improve patient care and outcomes through systematic review of care against explicit criteria and the implementation of change. Aspects of the structure, processes and outcomes of care are selected and systematically evaluated against explicit criteria. Where indicated, changes are implemented at an individual, team, or service level and further monitoring is used to confirm improvement in healthcare delivery.* ' (Principles for Best Practice in Clinical Audit, NICE, 2002)

Audit and Research thus both:
- involve answering specific questions which relate to the quality of care.
- can be carried out either prospectively or retrospectively.
- both audit and research involve sampling, questionnaires, data collection and analysis.

Research is:
- about creating new knowledge,
- about whether new treatments work better than established treatments
- whether some treatments are better than others.
- **It determines what is best practice**

Clinical audit is:
- a way of finding out if we are doing what we should be doing.
- are we following guidelines,
- **are we using best practice?**

The following points should help decide if the project is clinical audit or if it is research:
- Research creates new knowledge about what works and what is best; clinical audit tells us if we are following best practice.

- Research is based on a hypothesis; clinical audit measures against standards.
- Research can involve patients trying an untested treatment method; clinical audit **never** involves patients trying new treatment methods.
- Research may involve a degree of experimentation on patients; clinical audit **never** involves anything happening to the patient which is different to their normal treatment.
- One can't survive without the other. To be completely effective research can't survive without audit as we wouldn't know whether best practice was being carried out, and audit can't survive without research as without research we wouldn't know what best practice was! Research identifies areas for clinical audit and clinical audit identifies areas for research.

Clinical governance is defined as "A framework through which NHS organisations are accountable for continuously improving the quality of their services and safe-guarding high standards of care by creating an environment in which excellence in clinical care will flourish."

It's often thought of in terms of **the seven pillars** of clinical governance:
- clinical effectiveness,
- risk management,
- patient experience and involvement,
- communication,
- resource effectiveness,
- strategic effectiveness,
- learning effectiveness.

In short, it's **doing the right thing, at the right time, by the right person**—the application of the best evidence to a patient's problem, in the way the patient wishes, by an appropriately trained and resourced individual or team. But that's not all—that individual or team must work within an organisation that is accountable for the actions of its staff, values its staff (appraises and develops them), minimise risks, and learns from good practice, and indeed mistakes. (REFERENCE BMJ CAREERS)

EXPLAINING A DIAGNOSIS OF SUPRAVENTRICULAR TACHYCARDIA TO AN UPSET MOTHER

Information given to the candidate

You are a Paediatric Registrar in a District General Hospital. Jack is a 1-year-old child who presented with supraventricular tachycardia (SVT) which resolved after his face was dipped in ice cold water. Jack is now stable. His mother Ms Anderson was present while this was undertaken and is upset that as no one has spoken to her since arriving in the A&E.

Please speak to Ms Anderson, explain to her about SVT and the treatment strategy undertaken.

You are not expected to gather any further medical history but answer any queries that may arise during the discussion.

You have 9 minutes to complete the station; a warning bell will be given at 7 minutes (DR).

Information available to the mother (actor)

You are Ms Anderson, mother of 1-year-old Jack. Jack was unwell and not feeding well since yesterday. You brought him to A&E. The doctors took Jack and dipped the face in cold water which has frightened you. Though Jack is fine you are not sure what is going on as no one has talked to you.

You feel angry and helpless and would like to know what is going on? You have questions on the diagnosis and management? You want to know why other methods were not attempted as you felt dipping a child's face in water is cruel?

You expect an apology and reassurance that Jack is fine now. When the doctor explains that Jack had a problem when his heart was beating very fast and this made Jack feeling unwell. You also want to know whether this may recur again in the future. You have got two other children and are now scared that this may happen to your other children.

You are expected to exhibit controlled emotions. You are not expected to give any other personal information about yourself or your social life.

What is expected from the candidate?

- Introduces self to the mother and reassures child is now stable.
- Refers to actor as Ms Anderson and not as mum or mother.
- Addresses the child by his name 'Jack'
- Offers apologies for being unable to come and speak earlier as were busy treating Jack.

- Explains that Jack had SVT which happens when the heart beats very fast.
- Finds about Ms Anderson's understanding about SVT
- Mentions that the record showing tracing of the heart known as 'ECG' has confirmed the diagnosis.
- Explains that applying cold stimulus to face is an established practice and is known to work in SVT. Mentions that medicines are available to stop the SVT, however this needs more invasive and painful procedure. An intravenous line has to be inserted and medicines given that are not without its own risk.
- Clearly explains that this may happen again and Jack will need to assessed by a doctor.
- Explains that it is unlikely to occur in the other 2 siblings and offers screening for the family by ECG.
- Makes a clear plan for immediate management by monitoring Jack in the children's ward with a heart monitor being attached.
- Mentions that Jack will have further investigations and may need regular medicines.
- What further tests—should have a working knowledge.
- Does not gather further history or unnecessary information
- Summarises the discussion and addresses any concern raised by the mother
- **Checks mother understanding frequently—can ask her to recap what has been discussed.**
- Does not use medical jargon

NOTE

Explanation given to the mother. When heart is beating very fast, as was happening to Jack, it does not pump blood efficiently and that is why he was feeling unwell.

Further tests could be:
- ECG to look for Delta waves.
- 24 hour ECG or a 7-day event recorder.
- Echocardiogram to ensure normal anatomy – non-urgent.
- Treatment will depend on frequency of attacks and will need Paediatric cardiology advice.
  - β-blockers
  - Ablation of accessory pathway.

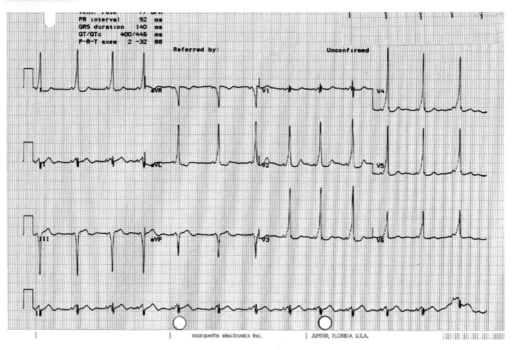

Fig. 7: ECG showing features of WPW syndrome

Note: Delta wave – slurring of R wave Lead I, V$_2$, V$_3$, V$_4$

Absence of r wave in V$_6$

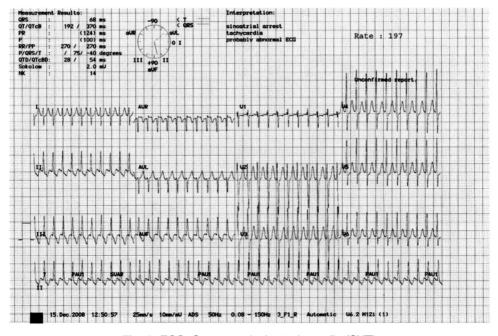

Fig. 8: ECG: Supraventricular tachycardia (SVT)

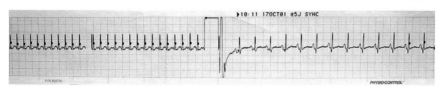

Fig. 9: Post conversion DC shock

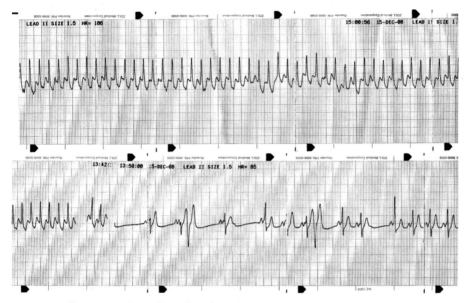

Figs 10 and 11: Post IV adenosine—conversion to sinus rhythm

SVT in children can be present at (or even before) birth with evidence of congestive heart failure. Newborns tolerate SVT episodes worse than older children and can decompensate fairly quickly. They present with poor feeding, pale and with peripheral shut down. On examination besides tachycardia and evidence of low cardiac output they may have significant hepatomegaly that can be easily missed. Treatment is cardioversion.

Some predisposing factors, such as Wolff-Parkinson-White syndrome may, rarely, run in families with otherwise normal hearts. They can occur with some forms of heart defect, such as Ebstein's anomaly.

Some types of SVT only occur after heart surgery, particularly after operations, like the Fontan, that change the way blood circulates within the heart.

Re-entry SVT

Re-entry SVT happens when the normal impulse from the atria to the ventricles returns back to the atria via an additional (abnormal) pathway. This creates a

circular movement of electrical impulses from atria to ventricles to atria …
and so on. This causes the heart to race quite suddenly for seconds, minutes or
hours.

a. **Accessory pathway SVT**

The common form of re-entry SVT is caused by an extra pathway in the heart
that is separate from the normal electrical pathway. If the extra pathway shows
up on ECG (electrocardiogram) while the child is resting it is known as Wolff-
Parkinson-White syndrome. In many others, the accessory pathway can only
be seen on an ECG during an attack of tachycardia.

b. **AV nodal tachycardia**

This less common form of re-entry tachycardia is not usually found in very
young children. It is due to an additional pathway in the AV node itself. This
form of tachycardia is not easy to recognise on an ECG.

Atrial tachycardia

Occasionally a tiny spot within the atria decides to produce very rapid impulses,
which are faster than the normal rhythm. This can start and stop at unpredictable
intervals. If the attacks continue for long periods of time, and it is not treated,
the heart muscle can be weakened. A fast form of this is known as atrial flutter,
and this is especially common after heart surgery.

Treatment

You or the older child must know what to do in the case of an attack – some
babies go back into a normal rhythm if a wet cold towel is wrapped around their
heads. Older children may be able to stop it with a cold fizzy drink, by making
their ears pop, or by taking slow deep breaths.

Radiofrequency ablation

For older children with an accessory pathway, who need to be on medication for
the foreseeable future, there may be the chance of cutting through the extra circuit.
It involves a catheter, a fine tube, being inserted into a vein and up to the heart
where it identifies the pathway. This is then destroyed using radio- frequency.

References

http://www.chfed.org.uk/information/heart conditions/
supraventricular tachycardia svt
http://medind.nic.in/icb/t05/i7/icbt05i7p609.pdf
http://www.emedicinehealth.com/supraventricular_tachycardia/
article_em.htm

EXPLAINING DIAGNOSIS OF FEBRILE CONVULSION TO AN ANXIOUS FATHER

Information given to the candidate

You are the paediatric registrar doing the ward round. Samuel is a 1-year- old boy who was brought to A&E by ambulance last night after having a generalised tonic clonic seizure associated with a fever of 39°C; this lasted for 2 minutes. Samuel was post-ictal for 10 minutes but has now recovered very well. A diagnosis of typical febrile convulsion is made and tonsillitis was found as the focus. Samuel has been commenced on oral penicillin. Samuel is now ready for discharge and you will be talking to his father Mr Julian Scott. Father has few questions which you will need to address during the discussion.

You are to speak to Samuel's father regarding his concerns.

You are not expected to gather any further medical history but answer any queries that may arise during the discussion.

You have 9 minutes to complete the station; a warning bell will be given at 7 minutes (DR).

Information available to the father (actor)

You are Mr Julian Scott, father of Samuel. Samuel had a fit last night with fever. Samuel looked pale and listless during the episode and you felt he was going to die. There is no family history of epilepsy but you recently came across a colleague whose child was diagnosed with a brain tumour after a fit. You want a brain scan to be done for Samuel as you feel that will rule out a brain tumour.

After having explained about febrile convulsion you feel a bit relaxed. You now want to know why this happened and whether this will happen again. You also want to know whether this could be epilepsy or whether Samuel needs any epilepsy medicines. You should be told by the candidate what to do in the event this happens again.

You are expected to exhibit controlled emotions. You are not expected to give any other personal information about yourself or Samuel.

What is expected from the candidate?

- Introduces self to the father and informs about the well-being of the child. Can take a lead from how he replies as how to address him?
- Refers to the actor/role player – as Mr Scott or Julian and not as dad or father.
- Addresses the child by his name 'Samuel'
- Explains and *agree* the agenda for the discussion

- Empathises with father that this was a difficult situation for him to see child fitting
- Reassures that this will not have long term effects for Samuel
- Clearly explains that this is febrile convulsion and not brain tumour.
- Candidate should not agree for a brain scan and need to explain why this is not necessary.
- Also explain that the one-third of children will have recurrence of a febrile seizure
- **Checks father understands about Samuel's diagnosis and reassures father that has not caused any brain damage and this is not epilepsy.**
- Explains that Samuel does not need any medicine.
- Also explains that Samuel will grow out of this and has a good prognosis.
- Gives a clear management plan that in future seizures Samuel needs to be put in a safe position and call an ambulance if lasts for >5 minutes.
- Does not gather further history or unnecessary information
- Summarises the discussion and addresses any other concerns raised by the father
- *Frequently checks father's understanding.*
- *Avoids monologue*—speak not for more than 30 seconds before checking understanding or seeking any questions.
- Does not use medical jargon

GENERAL NOTE

Febrile convulsion occurs typically in 6 months to 5 years of age in otherwise healthy children. This may occur without a high fever but need to demonstrate a fever soon after the episode. The fever should be extra-cranial in origin. In children <1 year of age a clear focus needs to be found, otherwise a full infection screen may be necessary. NICE guidelines clearly mentions that anti-pyretic such as Paracetamol does prevent a febrile convulsion. CT scan/EEG are not necessary in typical febrile convulsion and anti-epileptics should not be prescribed for febrile convulsion. One-third of children goes to develop recurrent febrile convulsions and all children grow out of it. <1% of children will develop epilepsy, this is the same as general population background risk.

CHILD PROTECTION—UNEXPLAINED HEAD INJURY

Information given to the candidate

You are the paediatric registrar working in the Paediatric Intensive Care unit. You are asked to speak to Ms Sandra James, mother of Jamie who is admitted in PICU. Jamie is a 6 weeks old boy who is ventilated with bilateral subdural haemorrhages. Neurosurgeons are involved and advised about conservative management.

Explain to Sandra about the finding of CT scans and further management

You are not expected to gather any further medical history but answer any queries that may arise during the discussion.

You have 9 minutes to complete the station; a warning bell will be given at 7 minutes (SE).

Information available to the mother (actor)

You are Ms Sandra James, a working mother with 3 young children. Child care is shared between yourself, the father and childminders. The children were bouncing on the bed and you heard a noise. When you arrived, you noticed that Jamie was lying on the floor. You called the ambulance immediately and came to the hospital. You are unable to explain how the head injury happened. You find it difficult to manage the family alone with three kids.

You are worried that the medical team may feel that you are an incompetent mother and social services will take your child away. You need to be reassured by the candidate that social services can also give support and can contribute by providing additional support.

You are expected to exhibit controlled emotions but are not supposed to volunteer any other information unless specifically asked.

What is expected from the candidate?
- Introduces self and clearly mentions aim for the discussion
- Exhibits empathy towards Jamie's condition
- Explains that Jamie is very sick and needs a ventilator for breathing but also reassures that he is currently stable and his condition is improving.
- ?Explains that the CT scan of brain showed that Jamie has blood outside his brain usually caused by some injury or fall. Can draw a diagram of the bleeding in relation to the brain and skull.
- ?Explain the advice received from the neurosurgeons.
- Also inform the mother that it is a standard protocol to inform the social services if any child is admitted to hospital with unexplained head injury.

- Inform mother about investigations like skeletal survey and ophthalmology examination to look for other injuries.
- Summarises the discussion and offers to speak to dad.
- *Frequently checks that mother understands.*
- *Avoids monologue*—speak not for more than 30 seconds before checking understanding or seeking any questions.
- Does not use medical jargon

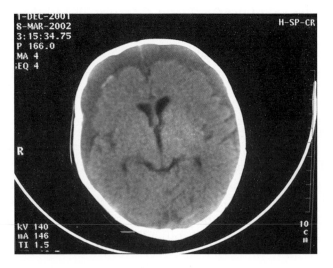

Fig. 12: CT scan of a 3-month-old boy admitted with nonspecific history and bruising on abdomen. Bilateral subdural haemorrhage

MEDICAL ETHICS/SPEAKING TO A NURSING COLLEAGUE

Information given to the candidate

You are the paediatric ST4 working in a District General Hospital. Natasha is a 3rd year nursing student attached to the department. The consultant has just finished and Natasha was present during the ward round. Jacob, a 13-year-old boy has just been diagnosed with leukaemia and his parents were informed by the Consultant separately with Jacob not present during the discussion. Jacob is going to the regional centre this afternoon for a bone marrow test and his parents requested that Jacob should not be told about the diagnosis prior to the bone marrow test.

Natasha has come to speak to you as she feels that Jacob should be told about the diagnosis straight away as he is Fraser competent to understand the nature of the problem.

Please speak to Natasha, explain why the team feels that parents wishes need to be respected and adhered to

You are not expected to discuss any more medical history but answer Natasha's queries and confusions that may arise during the discussion.

You have 9 minutes to complete the station; a warning bell will be given at 7 minutes (SP).

Information available to the nursing student (actor)

You are Natasha, a 3rd year nursing student doing your clinical posting in paediatrics. You are learning about the diseases in children and strongly feel that children should be involved in their diagnosis and the decision making process about their treatment. You do not understand why parents are obstructing the process and find it even more difficult why the medical team agreed to such a strange request.

Your younger brother had suffered from leukaemia at 8 years of age but is better now. He developed depression now and blamed your parents about not telling him the diagnosis and putting him through painful courses of chemotherapy. You feel that your brother is having low self esteem and poor quality of life not from the leukaemia but the process he went through.

After being explained about the domains of medical ethical framework for a difficult decision making process you understand why the medical team is withholding information. You expect to catch up to clarify your further doubts if offered the opportunity by the doctor.

You are expected to exhibit controlled emotions. You are not expected to give any other personal information about yourself or your social life.

What is expected from the candidate?

- Introduces self and clarifies about the agenda for the discussion, may tell that you have given the bleep to your colleague and is not going to be disturbed.
- Exhibits empathy towards a junior nursing colleague and enquires how she is finding her work in the department.
- Appreciates that Natasha feels strongly about the involvement of children in their management plan
- Tries to find why Natasha feels so strongly about involvement of Jacob in his diagnosis?
- Gives time to Natasha to express her feelings about her brother and gives a patient hearing
- Explains to Natasha about the 4 domains of medical ethical framework: autonomy (deliberate self rule), beneficence (try to do good), non-maleficience (avoid doing harm) and justice (patients and family to be treated as equal)
- Tries to explain to Natasha that it is a shock for the parents at this point and the team need to respect the parents' wishes of withholding the diagnosis from Jacob at present as every family has got their way of accepting a medical diagnosis.
- You thank Natasha for taking time to speak to you about her view points and request her to do some background reading about medical ethics.
- Summarises the discussion and offers to catch up with Natasha at a later date to clarify any further doubts.
- Avoids medical jargon

MEDICAL ETHICS AND GUIDING PRINCIPLES

Doctors and other healthcare professionals are constantly faced with situations requiring them to make decisions affecting other people. To choose the most appropriate course of action, reflecting on moral issues at work, the following principles can guide them.

The four Prima facie ethical principles that guide our moral path in dealing with any clinical situation are:

• Respect for autonomy

Voluntas aegroti suprema lex. patient has the right to refuse or choose their treatment. It is the moral obligation to respect the decision of another individual so far as the respect of that individual's wish is compatible with the respect of all others who may be affected by that decision. In Kantian terms "treat others as ends in themselves and never merely as means to an end" ie "do not use people as intermediaries to get something else". An example of autonomy is obtaining patients informed consent before doing anything to them. Medical confidentiality is an implication of respecting one's autonomy. Good communications is fundamental to our interactions to achieve the above.

• Beneficence and Non-maleficence

Salus aegroti suprema lex. A practitioner should act in the best interest of the patient. These two principles should be considered together. In the process of helping an individual, we always risk the possibility of harming them. We must always work towards producing a net benefit over any potential harm following our actions. Hippocratic moral obligation of medicine is to do net benefit with minimal harm. We must also help our patients to be more in control of their health needs and their ability to decide on options of treatments – Empowerment. Empowerment allows the obligation of beneficence and respect of autonomy to come together for a patient.

Primum non nocere. Non-maleficence is 'do no harm'—This overriding moral principle is vital to our dealing with all situations with a patient in our care and where harm is expected – it should be discussed and should be outweighed by the benefit from our action.

• Justice

Justice is synonymous with fairness. In healthcare this can be considered as: fair distribution of limited resources (Distributive justice); respect for people's rights (Rights based justice) and morally acceptable laws (Legal justice).
- *Double effect* refers to two types of consequences which may be produced by a single action, and in medical ethics it is usually regarded as the combined effect of beneficence and non-maleficence
- A commonly cited example of this phenomenon is the use of morphine or other analgesic in the dying patient. Such use of morphine can have the beneficial effect of easing the pain and suffering of the patient, while simultaneously having the maleficent effect of hastening the death of the patient through suppression of the respiratory system.

W D Ross, an English philosopher, introduced "Prima facie", meaning that the principle is binding unless it comes in conflict with another moral principle and if it does – then we have to choose between them.

The four principles do not provide a rigid algorithm that gives 'yes' 'no' answers at the end but give a framework and a common moral language for an individual to work their way through a situation—remembering that for most instances, there are no 'right' or 'wrong' decisions.

Raanan Gillon, visiting professor of medical ethics BMJ 1994;309:184-8

http://www.ncbi.nlm.nih.gov/pmc/articles/PMC2540719/pdf/bmj00449-0050.pdf

http://www.bma.org.uk/ethics/consent_and_capacity/childrentoolkit.jsp

EXPLAINING A DIAGNOSIS OF KAWASAKI'S DISEASE TO A MOTHER

Information given to the candidate

You are the paediatric registrar working in a District General Hospital. You are about to speak to Ms Emma Holden, mother of 2-year-old Jerome. Jerome has been diagnosed to have Kawasaki's disease. He does not have heart murmur and cardiac echocardiography has been arranged. The mother wanted to speak to someone about the Kawasaki's disease.

Discuss the diagnosis and management of Kawasaki's disease with her and explain what this means for Jerome

You are not expected to gather any further medical history but answer any queries that may arise during the discussion.

You have 9 minutes to complete the station; a warning bell will be given at 7 minutes (SE).

Information available to the mother (actor)

You are Ms Emma Holden, mother of 2-year-old Jerome. Jerome was unwell with a very high fever for 5 days. You have visited the A&E on 2 occasions to get Jerome checked over and were sent home with a diagnosis of viral infection. You are upset that Jerome has now been diagnosed with Kawasaki's disease. You were told about the diagnosis and were informed that he needs aspirin for his heart.

You want to know what Kawasaki disease is and what cause it? You also want to know whether it is contagious as you have 2 other young children. You also want to know why it was not diagnosed when you attended the A&E on two earlier occasions. You are worried about his heart and want to know more about it. You have been told by your doctor earlier that aspirin is not safe for children and why the doctors want to give it to Jerome.

You are expected to exhibit controlled emotions. You are not expected to give any other personal information about yourself or your social life.

What is expected from the candidate?
- Introduces self to the mother.
- Refers the actor as Ms Holden or Emma and not as mum or mother.
- Addresses the child by his name Jerome
- Checks mother understands about Jerome's diagnosis.
- Explains that Kawasaki is a clinical condition which causes inflammation of various tissues of the body like hands, legs, whites of eyes, lips, mouth and throat. It is not very clear what causes Kawasaki's disease.

- It is not contagious or hereditary in nature.
- Also explains that Kawasaki's disease is diagnosed on clinical symptoms as there is no test to confirm the diagnosis.
- Candidate should be able to tell mother about the diagnostic criteria for Kawasaki's disease.
- The primary concern with Kawasaki disease is the involvement of the heart and the blood vessels supplying the heart (coronary arteries).
- Kawasaki's disease can weaken the wall of one or more blood vessels supplying the heart, causing it to bulge or balloon out called 'aneurysm'
- On rare occasions, the aneurysm can also burst.
- The illness may also cause the heart muscle (myocardium) to be irritated and inflamed, as well as the membrane covering the heart (pericardium). Irregular heart rhythms and heart valve problems may also occur with Kawasaki's disease.
- In most cases, the effects on the heart caused by Kawasaki's disease are temporary, and resolve within five or six weeks. However, coronary artery problems may sometimes persist for longer periods of time.
- Explains the role of intravenous gamma globulin and aspirin to help decrease the swelling or inflammation that the illness produces as well as to prevent the formation of clots.
- Explains that aspirin is necessary here to prevent clot formation and close monitoring will be necessary. Reassures that aspirin is particularly unsafe in chickenpox. Explain that Cardiac echocardiogram is requested to look at heart and blood vessels. It needs to be repeated in 3–4 weeks time.
- Gives a clear management plan and follow-up plans
- Does not gather further history or unnecessary information
- Does not give false reassurance that Heart is not affected as there is no murmur heard
- Summarises the discussion and addresses any concern raised by the mother
- *Frequently checks mother's understanding.*
- *Avoids monologue*—speak not for more than 30 seconds before checking understanding or seeking any questions.
- Does not use medical jargon.

NOTE

Peeling of skin 2–3 weeks later is a characterstic feature.

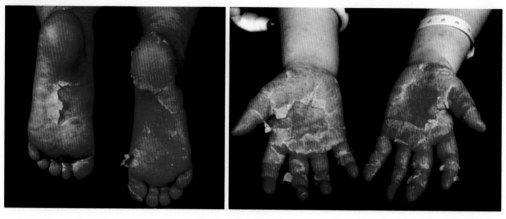

Fig. 13

Kawasaki Disease: Mucocutaneous lymph node syndrome; Infantile polyarteritis

Most patients are younger than age 5. The disease occurs more often in boys than in girls.

It may be an autoimmune disorder. The disorder affects the mucus membranes, lymph nodes, walls of the blood vessels, and the heart.

Disease begins with a high and persistent fever greater than 102°F, often as high as 104°F. A persistent fever lasting at least 5 days is considered a classic sign. The fever does not usually respond to normal doses of paracetamol or ibuprofen.

Five features including fever are necessary for a diagnosis. Other symptoms may include:

- Irritability
- Nonpurulent conjunctivitis
- Bright red, chapped, or cracked lips
- Red mucous membranes in the mouth
- Strawberry tongue, white coating on the tongue, or prominent red bumps on the back of the tongue
- Red palms of the hands and the soles of the feet
- Swollen hands and feet
- Skin rashes on the middle of the body, *not* blister-like
- Peeling skin in the genital area, hands, and feet (especially around the nails, palms, and soles)
- Swollen lymph nodes (frequently only one lymph node is swollen), particularly in the neck area
- Joint pain and swelling, frequently on both sides of the body
- Abdominal pain and diarrhoea

No tests specifically diagnose Kawasaki disease. The diagnosis is usually made based on the patient having most of the classic symptoms.

Atypical Kawasaki disease may be diagnosed in absence of classical signs and symptoms. Therefore, all children with fever lasting more than 5 days should be evaluated, with Kawasaki disease considered as a possibility.

Early treatment is essential for those who do have the disease.

The following tests are performed:

- Chest X-ray
- Complete blood count
- C-reactive protein (CRP)
- Echocardiogram
- Electrocardiogram
- ESR
- Serum albumin
- Serum transaminase
- Urinalysis—may show pus in the urine or protein in the urine

Investigations may reveal signs of myocarditis, pericarditis, arthritis, aseptic meningitis, and inflammation of the coronary arteries.

Children with Kawasaki disease are admitted to the hospital. Treatment must be started as soon as the diagnosis is made to prevent damage to the coronary arteries and heart.

Intravenous gamma globulin is the standard treatment. It is given in high doses. The child's condition usually greatly improves within 24 hours of treatment with IV gamma globulin.

High-dose aspirin is often given along with IV gamma globulin.

Even when they are treated with aspirin and IV gamma globulin, up to 25% of children may still develop problems in their coronary arteries.

Some research has suggested that adding steroids to the usual treatment routine may improve a child's outcome, but more research is needed.

With early recognition and treatment, full recovery can be expected. However, about 1% of patients die from complications of coronary blood vessel inflammation. Patients who have had Kawasaki disease should have an echocardiogram every 1–2 years to screen for heart problems.

Complications involving the heart, including vessel inflammation and aneurysm, can cause a heart attack at a young age or later in life.
http://www.ncbi.nlm.nih.gov/pubmedhealth/PMH0001984/

ANXIOUS MOTHER OF A PREMATURE BABY

Information given to the candidate: You are the Paediatric ST4 working in a District General Hospital. You are posted in the Special Care Baby Unit today. You have just reviewed Jacob who was born at 28 weeks, now 4 weeks old. He is the first child of the parents. He was doing well and was established on full enteral feeding. He developed Necrotising enterocolitis at 15 days of age. He was managed conservatively with intravenous antibiotics and total parenteral nutrition.

He is now recovered and ready to be commenced on enteral feeding. His mother, Mrs Sarah Thompson is extremely anxious about the feeds being restarted. She does not feel comfortable with it and wants to speak to a doctor.

Please speak to Jacob's mother and answer her questions.

You are not expected to gather any further medical history but answer any queries that may arise during the discussion.

You have 9 minutes to complete the station; a warning bell will be given at 7 minutes (NM).

Information available to the mother (actor)

You are Mrs Sarah Thompson and Jacob is your first child. Jacob was born at 28 weeks and this came as a big shock for you both (parents). As Jacob was fully established on feeds, you felt relaxed that he is out of the danger zone. Jacob then developed Necrotising Enterocolitis. He was nasogastric tube fed with your breast milk and nursed in a low dependency room when this happened.

He was moved back to the intensive care room and kept nil by mouth for 10 days. The nurse looking after Jacob has informed you that nasogastric tube feeds were going to be restarted.

You are worried that Necrotising Enterocolitis might recur when feeds are restarted. You are also concerned that Jacob might be moved back to the low dependency room too early and would not have adequate monitoring.

You had been expressing breast milk for Jacob earlier but now your milk supply is decreased. You are not comfortable with the idea of formula feeds as you have read in the internet that it might be one of the factors involved in necrotising enterocolitis.

You are expected to exhibit controlled emotions. You are not expected to give any other personal information about yourself or your social life.

What is expected from the candidate?

- Introduces self to the mother.
- Refers the actor as Ms Thompson or Sarah and not as mum or mother.
- Addresses the child by his name Jacob.
- Checks mother understands about Jacob's diagnosis (necrotising enterocolitis) and offers reassurance that Jacob is better now and you have just reviewed him in the ward round.
- Clearly mentions that as Jacob is now well this will be the right time to reintroduce the enteral feeds and that it will be done slowly with close monitoring.
- Shows empathy as it was both anxious and stressful period for the family.
- Explains that necrotising enterocolitis is a serious illness which mostly tends to affect babies who are born prematurely. The tissues in the gut can become swollen/inflamed and start to die. This can lead to a perforation (hole) developing which allows the contents of the gut to leak into the tummy. This can cause a very dangerous infection.
- Reassures mother that Jacob will not be transferred to the special care room till he fully established on enteral feeds again.
- Gives a clear management plan and follow-up plans
- Does not gather further history or unnecessary information
- Does not give false reassurance that NEC is not going to recur again but explains that close monitoring will be done when feeds are introduced and even thereafter.
- Offers to speak to the General Practitioner about medicines to enhance breast milk supply or use donor breast milk supply in the interim period.
- Summarises the discussion and addresses any concern raised by the mother
- *Frequently checks mother understands.*
- *Avoids monologue*—speak not for more than 30 seconds before checking understanding or seeking any questions.
- Does not use medical jargon

NOTE

Necrotising Enterocolitis: Risk factors

- Absent or reversed end diastolic flow on antenatal scan
- Prematurity.
- Birth asphyxia
- Hyperosmolar feeds—breast milk has protective effects

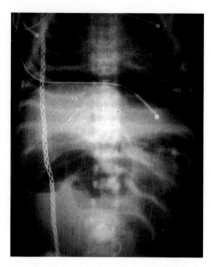

Fig.14: X-ray showing distended intestinal loops, free gas in abdomen under diaphragm plus a fluid level

- X-ray changes: Intestinal wall thickening—intra-mural gas – perforation – intra-peritoneal gas.

NEWBORN SCREENING—DISCUSSION WITH MEDICAL STUDENT

Information given to the candidate

You are the Paediatric ST4 in a District General Hospital. You have just finished the morning ward round in the Special Care Baby Unit. Charles, is a fourth year medical student doing his paediatric posting has accompanied you during the rounds. He has noticed one of the nurses requested the SHO for bloods from a baby for 'newborn blood spot screening test'.

Charles is very keen to know more about it. He has heard about it but does not quite understand what it is and why it is required. You oblige and speak to him about it in the doctor's office.

You have 9 minutes to complete the station; a warning bell will be given at 7 minutes (NM).

Information available to the medical student (actor)

You are Charles Henning, a fourth year medical student posted in the paediatric department. You have enjoyed the paediatric posting and is keen to learn more about neonates as you found it fascinating. You have heard about Newborn blood spot screening test but do not know what it means or constitutes of. You are also eager to know why the screening tests are done.

As you are explained this is a national programme and every baby born in the country gets it done you become more curious. You will want to know what happens if the results were to come back as positive. Does that mean the child has got the disease and will the baby need a repeat sample?

You also want to know about any special circumstances when a repeat sample will be necessary. This you will ask only when your previous queries have been adequately addressed.

Being a medical student you do understand medical terms however complex terms will need a simpler explanation for you level of expertise and understanding.

What is expected from the candidate?
- Introduces self and clearly mentions aim for the discussion
- Appreciates Charles' keenness to learn more about common paediatric issues.
- Finds about prior knowledge on the topic from Charles
- Mentions that screening tests are done generally by a heel prick blood sample at day 5 of age. Day 5 has been chosen as most babies will be established on milk feeds by then.

- The aim is to identify those babies who may be suffering from a number of different conditions – rare, but potentially serious. In most babies the results will be negative. In a small number of babies who are discovered to have one of the conditions, the benefits of screening at the earliest are enormous as it help in instituting early management with good outcome.
- Conditions tested at present are: phenylketonuria, congenital hypothyroidism, haemoglobinopathies (sickle cell disease, thalassemia), medium chain acyl carnitine dehydrogenase deficiency (MCAD), cystic fibrosis.
- Occasionally the babies may be need a second heel prick sample. This may be because enough blood was not collected, the result were unclear, or the baby was born early, not on milk feeds as baby may be unwell or had a blood transfusion.
- If the baby is thought to have one of the conditions, the family will be contacted and given an appointment with a specialist. Further diagnostic tests will be made to confirm the presence or absence of the condition.
- Checks that Charles understands and the candidate may need to go back if the student is not clear. Summarises the discussion and offers to catch up with Charles at a later date once he has done some more reading on the topic.
- *Avoids monologue*—speak not for more than 30 seconds before checking understanding or seeking any questions.
- Does not use medical jargon—*but* **should use adequate medical terminology as is** *speaking* **to a** *medical student*.
- Too much lay talk is not expected and can be counterproductive.

NEONATAL PAIN—DISCUSSION WITH F1 DOC

Information given to the candidate

You are going to see Anu, a new SHO in the department. She has been very troubled by crying newborn babies, more so when she has to take blood or put up iv infusion. She has asked to see you after the round in neonatal unit.

Your task is to speak to Anu and address her concerns
You are expected to address Anu's concerns, do not gather any more history but may answer any queries that Anu may raise during the discussion.

You have 9 minutes to complete the station; a warning bell will be given at 7 minutes (AG).

Information available to mother (actor)

You are Anu, a new F2/SHO in paediatrics. You like children and have always wanted to look after them. You have been in paediatrics for 1 month and in neonatal unit for 1 week. You are very upset by crying babies and want to know what can be done to be 'kind' to them.

• Why do we make babies cry?
• What pain killers can we give them?
• Why do not we always give them pain killers?
• How can we assess the pains babies are suffering?
• What strategies are available to deal with pain in babies?
• What medications are available?
• Opioid analgesia: Sucrose—does it really work? What evidence do we have?
• Paracetamol

What is expected from the candidate?

Examiners/Observers

• Appropriate greeting
• Arranges for a quiet room.
• Sympathetic and seeks other information about feeling of Anu, the SHO
• Information about previous knowledge. What she feels?
• Gives adequate information
• Acknowledge ignorance and to check up and meet again.
• Summarizes at the end

NOTE

Use of sucrose in 'pain' control of newborns undergoing traumatic procedure.

ADDISON'S DISEASE: DISCUSSION WITH NEW DIAGNOSED GIRL

Information given to the candidate: You are the paediatric ST3 working in a District General Hospital. Danielle Jones, 12-year-old was admitted with increasing lethargy and dizzy spells. She has been confirmed to have Addison's disease and is ready to be discharged on replacement therapy of glucocorticoids and mineralocortocoids.You are about to speak to Miss Danielle Jones, a 13 year old girl with Addison's disease.

Discuss with her diagnosis, medications, precautions and advice she will need.

You are not expected to gather any more history but may answer any queries that Danielle may raise during the discussion.

You have 9 minutes to complete the station; a warning bell will be given at 7 minutes (AG).

Information available to Miss Danielle Jones (actress/patient)
You are Miss Danielle Jones, 13 years old girl. You came to hospital as you felt tired and dizzy for few months. You have had lots of blood test and you are not too keen on 'needle picks'. You do feel better after the medicines doctors have given you. You do not like to take regular medicines and have a few questions you want to ask.

Your mother has been told that you have a condition called 'Addison's disease'.

• You want to know what is wrong with you
• What does it mean for you?
• Why do you have to take medicines for a long time?
• Why is it you? Why did it happen?
• People become hairy and big on steroids – Will you?

If it is *not* mentioned:

• Ask about medications to take if you are unwell on holiday.
• Steroid alert card
• Medi-alert bracelet

You need not volunteer any other information unless specifically asked.

What is expected from the candidate?
• Introduces self to Danielle.
• Explains the agenda/reason for meeting
• Clarify roles and identify topics to discuss
• Mentions the result and implications
• Checks Danille's understanding about the results and offers a simple explanation about the disease condition—Addison's disease.

- Explains role of steroids and replacement therapy.
- Glucocorticoids and mineralocorticoids
- Need for increase dosage when unwell
- Advice on Steroid card/Medi-Alert bracelet or necklace
- Does not make up side effects (if not known) but offers to consult a book and inform Danielle during the next discussion session.
- Agrees to come back when mother is present.
- Does not gather further history or unnecessary information
- Summarises the discussion and addresses any concern raised by Danielle
- Agrees to arrange for further discussion and mentions about information leaflets.
- *Avoids monologue*—**speak not for more than 30 seconds before checking understanding or seeking any questions.**
- Does not use medical jargon

NOTE

Addison's Disease

- Is most often caused by autoimmune disease and can be associated with other autoimmune disease processes
- Symptoms can be vague and wide ranging but hyperpigmentation and postural hypotension are significant signs.
- Investigations include U&Es, blood glucose, FBC, calcium
- Short and long ACTH stimulation tests
- Treatment involves long-term glucocorticoid and mineralocorticoid (hormones) replacement therapy.
- Steroids need to be increased during times of stress, illness, surgery.
- Need regular follow up for other disease.
- Polyglandular: There is a tendency for some disorders to occur together. For descriptive purposes, these are termed polyendocrine type I, type II and type III.
- Type I tends to begin in early childhood with skin infection (candidiasis) and is commonly associated with hypoparathyroidism as well as Addison's disease and is often associated with gonadal failure.
- Type II usually involves diabetes or thyroid disease and Addison's disease and sometimes ovarian failure and other non-endocrine autoimmune diseases.
- Type III involves thyroid autoimmune disease and at least two other autoimmune diseases, but not Addison's disease.
- Alert card: Necklace or bracelet by Medi-Alert and Steroid Alert Card.

Clinical Stations

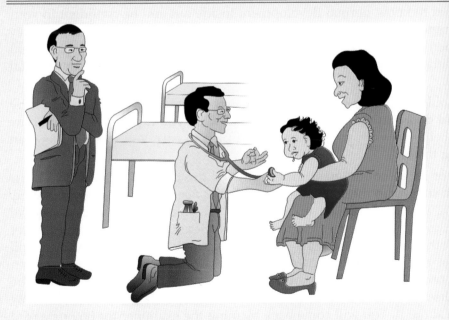

Clinical stations are about testing your competence in developing a rapport, examining a child, developing a clinical picture and then being able to discuss with the examiner the differential diagnosis and management. You are expected to be able to examine the child and would fail if you could not do that appropriately or even worse were 'rough' with the child however the main marks come in the discussion.

Your examination technique should be 'practiced' and 'sleek'. You should be able to finish a complete exam in 3–4 minutes. If you are taking longer during the preparation stage, i.e. now then you **need to practice more**. You should appear comfortable while examining a child and it should be obvious to the examiner that you have done this repeatedly during your training and is now your routine clinical practice.

There are six clinical stations: CVS, neurology and development are virtually a must, respiratory, abdomen, musculo-skeletal, **'Other'** offer other systems. In my experience candidates find CVS and neuro-developmental generally more difficult to master.

You need to know normal development inside out and be confident in your CVS examination. Candidates usually grade murmurs to be louder than they are and then get stuck with differential diagnosis. You need to be able to present your findings succinctly and this should usually lead to a logical differential diagnosis.

You should be prepared to discuss the investigations and **mentioning why you would do a particular investigation and what you expect to find** and how that will help you with your management plan to earn you more marks than just listing them.

Think of three commonest diagnoses for the clinical findings. In your discussion start with the commonest and do not need to proceed beyond three. Presuming you have picked up the correct physical signs, made a logical deduction and given logical differential, you will be asked how to proceed further to confirm the diagnosis and what the management would be. Rarely, there will be time for more than this. However, if you start with diagnoses 6–7–8 from reference textbooks (which obviously will be rarer) then be sure you will be asked to discuss the condition 8, and I am reasonably certain that you will know very little about it. You will come back blaming the examiner for having asked you about this condition.

The examiners are not there to make your life harder, unbelievable as it may seem under the circumstances. You may be asked 'Are you sure?' They are not trying to trick you. During one exam a candidate examined a 6-year-old child with a harsh systolic murmur, 3/6, maximal at the left sternal border, difficult to be certain if it was maximal at the upper or lower sternal edge. It could also be heard on lateral left chest wall, but much softer. The differential diagnosis would be Pulmonary stenosis or VSD, and I would have accepted both, in either order. The candidate was good with the child, elicited the clinical signs and presented them well. "In conclusion this child has a VSD".

I asked if he was sure?

"Yes". "Can it be anything else?" "No, it is a classic murmur of a VSD". He did not pass the cardiovascular station!!

Do not be rough with a child. That is an *unacceptable*. If a child is not in a Co-operating mood usually due to being tired, do *not* coerce the child to go through the examination. The examiners have seen this number of times during their clinical practice and during the exam and are very much aware of the difficulty that may arise from this. There is a criteria in the mark sheet about an unco-operative child and your performance will be judged with due consideration. Upsetting the child will not endear you to the patient, the family or to the examiner.

Do not despair if you think you have 'bombed' a station. We are usually over critical of our performance. You might not have. Do not rely on the smile from the examiner – he may be smiling, pleased at your expert examination technique or he may be contemplating the end of your time with him because you have not met his expectation.

I teach to consider the exam as a 'cricket match' with each station being one wicket. You are the captain. Just because one wicket falls early does not mean the match is over and everything is lost. Keep your cool, each wicket is a fresh start and can help you recover the lost ground.

Remember—you have not failed until you have seen the letter from the RCPCH.

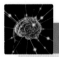

Remember !

Practice complete examination of one system per day in
every child you see.
Know 3 top diagnosis for common presentations in each system
Do not look for or rely on 'encouragement' during the exam.

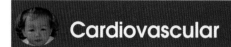

THIS STATION POSES UNDUE DIFFICULTY TO CANDIDATES PREPARE WELL

An Approach to A Child with A Murmur

Cardiac murmur: Innocent versus Pathological

It is important to understand the basic cardiac physiology and pressures during the cardiac cycle to be able to explain it. Do read on even if you know all about murmurs and have just completed a job in cardiology.

You need to be clear of *'What is a murmur? What causes a murmur?'*

I would take a ventricular septal defect of moderate size as an example to illustrate.

A murmur is caused by turbulence of blood by its passage through the heart or blood vessels. The turbulence can be due to the blood moving across a hole in the septum separating the two ventricles. It can also be caused by blood being forced out through the narrow valve or artery during systole or leaking through an incompetent valve during diastole.

Blood flows at the speed of about 1 meter/sec in the aorta. Normally it returns from the systemic circulation to the right side of the heart and is pumped to the lungs, similarly it returns to the left atrium and is pumped to the body by the left ventricle. The right side of the heart receives the same amount of blood as the left side.

Blood will flow from an area of high pressure to lower pressure. Hence if there is an opening between two chambers, i.e. left and right ventricle then the blood will flow from left ventricle to right ventricle as there is a pressure difference.

What is the pressure in the left ventricle?

Have a little think, if there is no aortic valve obstruction then the left ventricle peak pressure will be the systemic systolic pressure, 50 mmHg in a neonate and 120 mmHg in an adult.

What is the pressure in the right ventricle?

It is equal to the systemic pressure in utero and soon after birth. This is because right ventricle is pumping into descending aorta via the patent ductus arteriosus and has to match left ventricular pressure. After the first breath, lungs open with fall in pulmonary resistance and the pressure decreases gradually over the next few weeks to around 20 to 25 mmHg.

You may now be able to describe **why a newborn baby may not have an audible murmur soon after birth even though there is a hole between the two ventricles**. This is because the pressure in the right ventricle equals the pressure in the left ventricle and hence there is no flow of blood across the septal defect, there is no turbulence to cause the additional noise.

Over the next few days and weeks as the pressure in the left ventricle increases slightly and pressure in the right ventricle decreases significantly, blood start shunting from left to right causing a murmur.

Hence it is normal not to be able to pick up a ventricular septal defect murmur soon after birth. Symptoms of congestive failure may also be absent for the first few weeks after birth.

In stenosis of a valve or of artery, the blood being pushed out accelerates, and it is this increased velocity that causes turbulence and hence the murmur. Thus murmurs of Aortic or Pulmonary stenosis will be heard from day one.

In Tetralogy of Fallot (ToF), the murmur heard is of pulmonary stenosis and not of the blood flowing across the VSD.

In atrial septal defect (ASD), the blood flowing across from left atrium to right atrium is not against a high pressure difference (gradient) and thus does not cause the murmur. The murmur heard in ASD is due to increased blood flow across the pulmonary valve (systemic return + shunted blood across ASD) making it a 'relative' pulmonary stenosis. This systolic murmur, thus is never very loud – usually grade 2/6, with fixed splitting of 2nd sound, i.e. the interval between closure of aortic and pulmonary valve does not vary with respiration.

If the patient has a median sternotomy scar or any other significant sign suggestive of cardiac surgery, interpreting the aetiology of murmurs would be difficult, you will not be able to comment with confidence on the anatomical defect. A systolic murmur should be explained as a shunt, stenosis or valvular regurgitation. Also feel for brachial in both arms, in case they have been used in Blalock-Taussig or modified BT shunt.

Cardiac scenario and explaining to parents/role player is common.

Example of an explanation that may be used for **'What is an innocent/flow murmur?'**

Every heart makes noises when blood is pumped due to contracting of the heart, opening and closing of valves and blood being churned in the heart. Some individuals have an additional noise and that is what we call a murmur. It may be due to a narrowing of a valve or a blood vessel or there may be a hole in the heart. Sometimes it is due to just the way blood is flowing and is called an 'Innocent murmur' when there are no structural abnormalities.

I think of two facts when describing a murmur: Laminar flow and a jet of water.

Blood and water have similar characteristics when flowing. If you walk along a river, water flowing straight is quiet as is laminar. When is goes round a bend, it gets disturbed and makes a noise-turbulence.

Second is: sink tap, when the tap is half open, the water flowing does not make a noise but when opened fully and more water flowing it makes a noise. Nothing is wrong with the tap or the water except more water if flowing thorough the same size tube.

We can thus hear a murmur in a child who has fever, the heart pumps more blood, as it is needed by the body and if we listen then, a murmur may be heard that will not be there when the child is better.

Innocent murmurs are mostly: Soft, short, systolic, change with posture (sitting and lying down) and children are asymptomatic.

Common cause of Innocent or Flow Murmur are:
- Pulmonary flow murmur
- Venous hum (disappears with gentle pressure on jugular vein)
- Stills murmur (lower left sternal border, early systolic)

This understanding should help you explain your findings during the exam.

You may get a child with innocent murmur in the examination hence be prepared to comment on it being an innocent murmur and do not make it pathological.

There are other facts you need to brush up on.

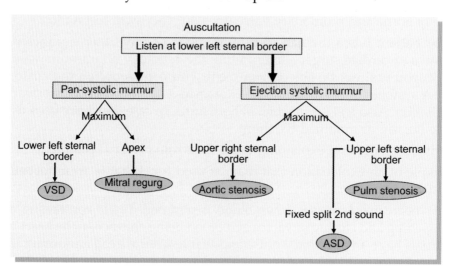

Fig. 15

How would you proceed with a patient in 'real' if the patient is not 'co-operating and does not perform/play ball'. This can happen for a number of reason, a tired child, bored child, hungry child. Do *not* lose your cool and panic. This is taken into consideration by the examiner when assessing your performance. There are columns in the mark sheet to say how many times the child has 'performed' before and if he/she are behaving appropriate for the situation.

You should have some distraction techniques up your sleeve. Some that I use are:

- Remain calm and smile. Remember children can sense 'nervousness'.
- Engage the child with a simple question: what is his favorite toy? What did he have to eat earlier? What does he like doing best?
- Examine a doll or a toy while talking to it.
- 'Pretend' to examine mother. Start with examining her leg, move up to the arm and then on to chest. Once the child feels a little secure, move over a place the stethoscope on his feet, move up gradually to his hands and after a few seconds gently move over to his precordium. Hopefully he would not have any clothes on his chest but if he does – then proceed to auscultate through his clothes. You will be able to get most of the auscultatory information through his clothes. Once you are reasonably satisfied ask his mother to remove his top clothes as inspection is mandatory part of any examination and can still be done even with a child who is a little upset. If the child remains playful, then after inspection you can have another attempt at listening to the heart.
- Engaging and distracting children is a core skill for paediatricians.

If even after your 'charm offensive' the child remains unimpressed and continues to be reluctant for a stranger to come close—*do not force* yourself on the child and *never* be *rough* with a *child*. This will be sure way to get *unacceptable* for the station.

You can score marks and pass the station by making sense of what you are able to observe, without necessarily auscultating the child.

You will be able to comment on your observations noting cardiac clues and other circumstantial clues.

- Left lateral thoracotomy scar suggestive of possible:
  - Blalock-Taussig shut (BT shunt)
  - Pulmonary artery banding
  - Coarctation of aorta repair
  - PDA ligation
- Central sternotomy scar: It is very difficult to guess the anatomical defect and surgery undertaken.
- 'Starry' back of hand: Suggestive of multiple attempts at IV drips.
- Oblong head, flattened side to side: Premature infant.
- Dysmorphic features suggestive of:
  - Down syndrome
  - Noonan's syndrome

- Di-George's syndrome
- Williams syndrome

Before concluding your examination of CVS:
- Always check femoral pulses
- Always feel for hepatomegaly
- Always listen to the back for murmur of coarctation
- Always check Blood Pressure or ask for it
- Always plot weight and height on appropriate chart or mention your intention.

After completing you examination pause for 30 seconds to pull the finding together, work through a differential diagnosis for *your* findings and *not* from the book you read. Think through of the logical *investigations* you will need to narrow your differential and confirm your diagnosis.

Think thorough what you would expect each of the investigations to reveal and how that would help you with your diagnosis. This will get you more marks then just giving a list and hoping the examiner knows what to expect from the list of investigations.

Common investigations are:

Blood pressure: Mention you will like to take BP to ensure it is normal (it is to be considered part of clinical examination.)

CXR: To look for cardiac shape and size, i.e. cardiomegaly and pulmonary plethora.

ECG: Rhythm, Left, Right or biventricular hypertrophy

Echocardiogram: Confirming anatomy. Identifying the defect. Good idea of function.

Holter 24 hour/longer term monitoring: Looking for arrhythmia, linking with symptom diary.

After you have presented your findings succinctly and lead into your diagnosis or differential diagnosis. You would have honed down to most likely diagnosis e.g. VSD, pulmonary stenosis, aortic stenosis.

Keep in mind that you are unlikely to get very ill children in the exam. VSD is common but a child in congestive failure with VSD will be rare, at least in UK. In overseas centers you can expect to see children with Rheumatic heart disease with mitral valvular murmur – stenosis and/or regurgitation. Children with conditions more advanced in their natural history. Un-operated congenital lesions.

It is important to be confident of clinical signs you have identified, place them in the cardiac cycle. You should be able to describe a murmur under:

- Location: Lower left sternal border, upper right sternal border
- Time in cardiac cycle and Grade: Ejection systolic, pan systolic, 3/6
- Radiation: Heard all over precordium, radiates into neck

You can score good marks by discussing appropriate management. This may include medication, possible surgery and discussion with parents.

CHILD WITH VSD

Information given to the candidate

You are the candidate and on entering the station, the examiner introduces you to a 5-year-old boy Jagan and his mother, both sitting on chair.

Jagan has come for a check as he was noted to have a murmur on school medical check. He looks well and is in shorts. You are requested to do a cardiovascular examination and any other relevant examination to reach a diagnosis.

You are allowed to talk to the patient but are not allowed to ask any history unless allowed by the examiner.

You have 9 minutes to complete the station; a warning bell will be given at 7 minutes (AG).

The examination

You introduce yourself to Jagan and his mother and obtain a verbal consent. You explain hand hygiene has been adhered to.

On general inspection
- There are no medicine or medical devices around him.
- Jagan is 'average size and built'
- He is comfortable, pink, not distressed.
- Chest is normal, normal respiratory rate
- No scars noted

General physical and system exam: Explain to Jagan what you will be doing
- No clubbing
- No cyanosis
- Brachial/radial pulse equal, 80/min, regular
- Precordium – no heave or thrill, apex 5th ICS and mid clavicular line
- Heart sounds: 1st and 2nd Normal.
- Harsh pan systolic murmur 3/6, maximal at lower left sternal area
- Does not change with posture
- No murmur heard at back
- Femoral pulses are easily palpable

You summarise your findings: You have examined Jagan, a 7-year-old boy. He is comfortable at rest. He is pink and seems appropriately grown, but would like to plot him on appropriate chart. There are no scars. He has no clubbing or cyanosis. He has regular pulse, 80/min. Peripheral pulses are easily palpable with no radio-femoral delay. Percordium feels normal with no heaves or thrill. Apex is in midcalvicular line, in 5th ICS. On auscultation there is a harsh pan systolic murmur grade 3/6, maximal in the lower left sternal area. His heart sounds 1st and 2nd are heard and are Normal. 2nd is not prominent. (*If you are sure of split sounds—then you can comment on it appropriately or skip it*). There are no bruits or murmurs in the neck or the back. "I would check his blood pressure."

You do not need to stop and can move on to your impression

In my opinion Jagan is well. My findings are consistent with a Ventricular Septal Defect. I would like to confirm that by investigations. The most useful will be an echocardiogram that will confirm anatomy and function. An ECG to check for rhythm and electrical activity. If Echocardiogram is not available I will also like to do a CXR to look for cardiac size and pulmonary plethora.

You should following this be prepared for discussion as the case is simple and you should have ample time left till the bell rings.

What is expected from the candidate?
- Introduces self to the mother and Jagan and requests verbal consent.
- Makes it known that hand hygiene has been done before touching the patient.
- Keeps the patient at ease and gives simple and easy to understand commands.
- Inspects and comments on observations.
- Comments absence of scars
- Follows logical sequence to cardiac examination
- Auscultates the back and neck
- Picks up normal heart sounds and murmur
- Works through and evaluates different pathologies
- The candidate should be able to correlate the findings and discuss aetiology and management.

NOTE
If you are asked "Can it be anything else?"

Do not take it as a trick—it may be you might be wrong and the examiner is trying to 'help' you reconsider. If you are sure then say you still think the most likely diagnosis is a VSD but will consider a differential including ...."

You should then come out with your differential: "Yes it could be and I would like to consider!: Pulmonary stenosis as the murmur is in the same area and possibly a VSD". These can be checked with an echocardiogram

Do not say "No it cannot be anything else" or "it is classic VSD, you are sure".

This attitude, if you are wrong, suggests you are inflexible and once have made up your mind, are not open to other suggestions. This can be disastrous on a ward.

In this scenario you will have time to score marks with your discussion. Prepare well and 'lead you discussion':

1. Current guidelines on bacterial endocarditis prophylaxis. In UK prophylaxis is not recommended.
2. Presentation in newborn period: in small or a large VSD
3. Medium to long term out come and need for follow up.

Picture of VSD on Colour Flow

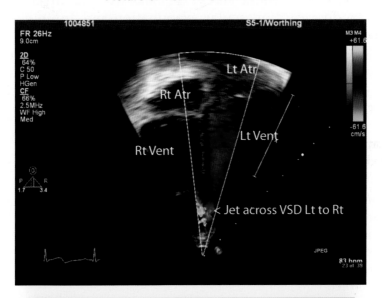

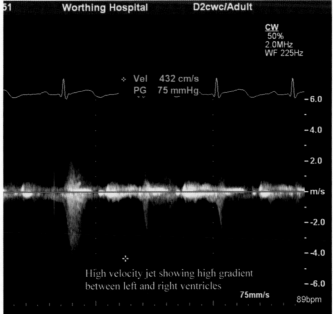

Figs 16 and 17: 4 chamber view with colour flow demonstrating Jet flow across ventricular septum

CHILD WITH ATRIAL SEPTAL DEFECT

Information given to the candidate

You are the candidate and on entering the station, the examiner introduces you to a 7-year-old boy Mohan and his mother, both sitting on chair.

Aaron has come for a routine check. He looks well and in shorts. You are requested to do a cardiovascular examination and any other relevant examination to reach a diagnosis.

You are allowed to talk to the patient but are not allowed to ask any history unless allowed by the examiner.

You have 9 minutes to complete the station; a warning bell will be given at 7 minutes. (AG)

The examination

You introduce yourself to Mohan and his mother and obtain a verbal consent. You explain hand hygiene has been adhered to:

On general inspection
• There are no medicine or medical devices around him.
• Mohan is 'average size and built'
• He is comfortable, pink, not distressed.
• Chest is normal, normal respiratory rate
• No scars noted

General physical and system exam
• No clubbing
• No cyanosis
• Brachial/radial pulse equal, 75 min, regular
• Precordium—no heave or thrill, apex 5th ICS and mid clavicular line
• Heart sounds: 1st and 2nd Normal. 2nd prominent, split, fixed splitting
• Ejection systolic murmur 2/6, maximal at upper left sternal area
• No murmur heard at back
• Femoral pulses are easily palpable

You summarise your findings: you have examined Mohan, a 7-year-old boy. He is comfortable at rest. He is pink and seems appropriately grown, but would like to plot him on appropriate chart. There are no scars. He has no clubbing or cyanosis. He has regular pulse; 75/min. Peripheral pulses are easily palpable with no radio-femoral delay. Precordium feels normal with no heaves or thrill. Apex is in mid calvicular line, in 5th ICS. On auscultation there is a systolic murmur grade 2/6, maximal in the upper left sternal area. His heart sounds 1st and 2nd are heard. 2nd seems prominent. It is split and I am not sure if it fixed split. (If you are sure of fixed split – then you can comment on it appropriately). There are no bruits or murmurs in the neck or the back. You will like check his blood pressure.

You do not need to stop and can move on to your impression: I think Mohan is well. My findings suggest he is most likely to have an ASD. I would like to confirm that by investigations. The most useful investigation will be an echocardiogram that will confirm anatomy and function. An ECG to check for rhythm and electrical activity, ASD quite often is associated with Partial right bundle branch block. If Echocardiogram is not easily available I will also like to do a CXR to look for cardiac size and pulmonary plethora. You should following this be prepared for discussion.

What is expected from the candidate?
- Introduces self to the mother and Mohan and requests verbal consent.
- Makes it known that hand hygiene has been done before touching the patient.
- Keeps the patient at ease and gives simple and easy to understand commands.
- Inspects and comments on observations.
- Comments absence of scars
- Follows logical sequence to cardiac examination
- Auscultates the back and neck
- Picks up 'different' heart sounds· Works through and concludes differential pathologies
- The candidate should be able to correlate the findings and discuss aetiology and management.

NOTE

If you are asked "Can it be anything else?"

Do not take it as a trick—it may be you might be wrong. You should then come out with your differential: "Yes it could be and I would like to consider!: Pulmonary stenosis as the murmur is in the same area and possibly a VSD". These can be checked with an echocardiogram

Do not say "No it cannot be anything else" or "it is classic ASD, you are sure".

Splitting of, fixed splitting and loud heart sounds. Normally there is a change in the timing of closure of aortic valve and pulmonary valve. This changes during inspiration and expiration, Split and varies versus in ASD when there is no variation in closure thus appearing to have the same gap between the two—Fixed splitting.

Movement of blood across atrial septal defect is from left to right, this does not cause the murmur. The murmur is caused by the blood flow across pulmonary valve and is unlikely to be louder than 2/6.

ASDs are now commonly closed by trans-catheter closing devices.

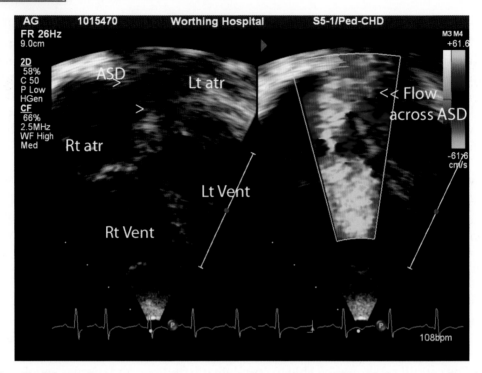

Fig. 18: Echocardiogram—colour flow mapping: Demonstrating ASD with flow across from left atrium to right atrium

CHILD WITH PROSTHETIC VALVE

Information given to the candidate

You are the candidate and on entering the station, the examiner introduces you to an 11-year-old boy Aaron and his mother, both sitting on chair.

Aaron has come for a routine check. He looks well and in shorts. You are requested to do a cardiovascular examination and any other relevant examination to reach a diagnosis.

You are allowed to talk to the patient but are not allowed to ask any history unless allowed by the examiner.

You have 9 minutes to complete the station; a warning bell will be given at 7 minutes. (AG)

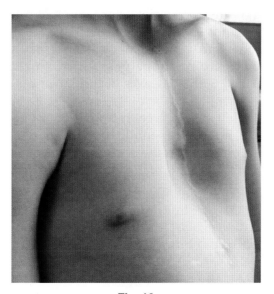

Fig. 19

The examination

You introduce yourself to Aaron and his mother and obtain a verbal consent. You explain hand hygiene has been adhered to:

On general inspection
- There are no medicine or medical devices around him.
- Aaron is 'average size and built'
- He is comfortable, pink, not distressed.
- Median sternotomy scar, normal skin colour, pale pink

- Pectus excavatum
- Two little scars upper abdominal area

General physical and system exam

- No clubbing
- No cyanosis
- Brachial/radial pulse equal, 75 min, regular
- Central scar not tender
- Precordium—no heave or thrill, apex 6th ICS and mid axillary line
- Heart sounds: Clicky noise heard, maximum. Upper right sternal area
- Pan systolic murmur 3/6 at lower left sternal area
- No murmur heard at back
- Femoral pulses are easily palpable

You summarise your findings: You have examined Aaron, an 11-year-old boy. He is comfortable at rest. He is pink and seems appropriately grown, but would like to plot him on appropriate chart. He had a median sternotomy scar, that is pale pink and 2 smaller scars in lower thoracic area. There is pectus excavatum. He has no clubbing or cyanosis. He has regular pulse; 75/min. Peripheral pulses are easily palpable with no radio-femoral delay. Precordium feels normal with no heaves or thrill. Apex is in anterior axillary line, in 6th ICS. On auscultation there is a loud systolic murmur grade 3/6, maximal in the lower left sternal area, heard all over precordium. His heart sounds are 'different'. They do not sound normal. They have a clicky character. There are no bruits or murmurs in the neck or the back. I will like to check his blood pressure to confirm it is normal.

You do not need to stop and can move on to your impression:

I think Aaron is well. My clinical findings suggest he has a VSD. Displaced apex beat suggest cardiomegaly. He also has 'different' sounding heart sounds that I have not heard before but I think they could be due to a mechanical artificial valve.

Pectus excavatum is due to cardiac surgery.

You should following this be prepared for discussion.

What is expected from the candidate?
- Introduces self to the mother and Aaron and requests verbal consent.
- Makes it known that hand hygiene has been done before touching the patient.
- Keeps the patient at ease and gives simple and easy to understand commands.
- Inspects and comments on observations.
- Comments on median scar, good candidate will also mention colour
- Follows logical sequence to cardiac examination

- Auscultates the back and neck
- Picks up 'different' heart sounds
- Works through and concludes two different pathologies
- The candidate should be able to correlate the findings and discuss aetiology and management.

NOTE

This patient has a small VSD. He also has a prosthetic Aortic valve. He had critical aortic stenosis and had balloon dilatation soon after birth. He suffered from residual stenosis and regurgitation of aortic valve leading to cardiomegaly. The valve was replaced a few months ago, as the scar has not 'healed' fully and changed colour as of an old scar. The two small scars are likely to be due to post operative 'drains'. He is currently on anticoagulants.

You should not be 'afraid' to mention any findings that are *not* normal. You have to be confident of what is Normal and are expected to be able to comment on 'abnormal signs'.

You may be invited by examiner to ask Aaron or his mother a question. You can then ask about "What was the surgery for?"

You should be able to discuss the prophylaxis and advice to Aaron.

CHILD WITH PULMONARY STENOSIS—NOONAN'S SYNDROME

Information given to the candidate

You are the candidate and on entering the station, the examiner introduces you to a 3-year-old boy Matthew and his mother, both sitting on chair. Matthew has come for a check as he was noted to have a murmur by his General Practitioner (GP). He looks well and in shorts. You are requested to do a cardiovascular examination and any other relevant examination to reach a diagnosis.

You are allowed to talk to the patient but are not allowed to ask any history unless allowed by the examiner.

You have 9 minutes to complete the station; a warning bell will be given at 7 minutes. (AG)

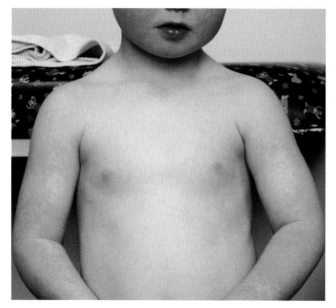

Fig. 20

The examination

You introduce yourself to Matthew and his mother and obtain a verbal consent. You explain hand hygiene has been adhered to:

On general inspection
• There are no medications or medical devices around.
• Matthew is 'average size and built'

- He is comfortable, pink, not distressed.
- Slight webbing of his neck
- His head looks a little large compared to his body
- Chest is normal, normal respiratory rate
- No scars noted

General physical and system exam: Explain to Matthew what you will be doing and notice his understanding is not as you will expect
- No clubbing
- No cyanosis
- Brachial/radial pulse equal, 80/min, regular
- Precordium—no heave or thrill, apex 5th ICS and mid clavicular line
- Heart sounds: 1st and 2nd Normal.
- Harsh pan systolic murmur 2/6, maximal at upper left sternal area
- Does not change with posture
- No murmur heard at back
- Femoral pulses are easily palpable

You summarise your findings: You have examined Matthew, a 3-year-old boy. He is comfortable at rest. He is pink and seems appropriately grown, but would like to plot him on appropriate chart. He has mild webbing of the neck and has soft dysmorphic features. His comprehension seems less than a child of his age. There are no scars. He has no clubbing or cyanosis. He has regular pulse; 80/min. Peripheral pulses are easily palpable with no radio-femoral delay. Precordium feels normal with no heaves or thrill. Apex is in mid calvicular line, in 5th ICS. On auscultation there is an ejection systolic murmur grade 2/6, maximal in the upper left sternal area. His heart sounds 1st and 2nd are heard and are Normal. 2nd heart sound is not prominent. (*If you are sure of split sounds—then you can comment on it appropriately or skip it*). There are no bruits or murmurs in the neck or the back. You will like to check his blood pressure.

You do not need to stop and can move on to your impression:

In my opinion Matthew is well. My findings are consistent with Pulmonary Stenosis. He also has features suggestive of Noonan's syndrome.

I would like to confirm that by investigations. The most useful will be an echocardiogram that will confirm anatomy and function. An ECG to check for rhythm and electrical activity. If echocardiogram is not available I will also like to do a CXR to look for cardiac size and pulmonary plethora.

For his Noonan's syndrome I will refer him to a geneticist for further advice and genetic testing.

You should following this be prepared for discussion as the case is simple and you should have ample time left till the bell rings.

What is expected from the candidate?
- Introduces self to the mother and Matthew and requests verbal consent.
- Makes it known that hand hygiene has been done before touching the patient.
- Keeps the patient at ease and gives simple and easy to understand commands.
- Inspects and comments on observations.
- Comments absence of scars
- Follows logical sequence to cardiac examination
- Auscultates the back and neck
- Picks up normal heart sounds and murmur
- Works through and evaluates different pathologies

The candidate should be able to correlate the findings and discuss aetiology and management.

NOTE

In this scenario you will have time to score marks with your discussion. Prepare well and 'lead you discussion'.

CHILD WITH REPAIRED COARCTATION OF AORTA

Information given to the candidate
You are the candidate and on entering the station, the examiner introduces you to 8-year-old boy John and his mother, both sitting on chair.

John has come for a check. He looks well and in shorts. You are requested to do a cardiovascular examination and any other relevant examination to reach a diagnosis.

You are allowed to talk to the patient but are not allowed to ask any history unless allowed by the examiner.

You have 9 minutes to complete the station; a warning bell will be given at 7 minutes. (AG)

The examination: You introduce yourself to John and his mother and obtain a verbal consent. You explain hand hygiene has been adhered to:

On general inspection
• There are no medicine or medical devices around him.
• John is 'average size and built'
• He is comfortable, pink, not distressed.
• Chest is normal, normal respiratory rate
• Scar from left mid axillary line to inferior border of scapula

General physical and system exam: Explain to Ram what you will be doing
• No clubbing
• No cyanosis
• Pulse 80/min, left brachial pulse is absent
• Precordium – no heave or thrill, apex 5th ICS and mid clavicular line
• Heart sounds: 1st and 2nd Normal.
• Ejection systolic murmur 2/6, maximal over upper right sternal area – no radiation
• Does not change with posture
• Femoral pulses are easily palpable

You summarise your findings: You have examined John, an 8-year-old boy. He is comfortable at rest. He is pink and seems appropriately grown, but would like to plot him on appropriate chart. There is a scar on left side of his chest, extending from left mid axillary line to inferior margin of scapula. It is dark pink in colour. He has no clubbing or cyanosis. He has regular pulse; 80/min. Left radial pulse is weakly palpable and left brachial is absent. Other peripheral pulses are easily palpable with no radio-femoral delay. Precordium feels normal with no heaves or thrill. Apex is in midclavicular line, in 5th ICS. On auscultation his heart sounds 1st and 2nd are heard and are Normal. 2nd is not prominent. (*If you are sure of split sounds—then you can comment on it appropriately or skip it*). There is an ejection systolic murmur grade 2/6, maximal in upper right sternal border. It does not radiate to the neck. There are no bruits or murmurs in the neck or the back. You will like to check his blood pressure.

You do not need to stop and can move on to your impression: In my opinion John is well. My most likely diagnosis is that he had coarctation of aorta that has been repaired using the subclavian artery with normal femoral pulses now. He also has a murmur suggestive of mild Aortic valve stenosis.

I would like to confirm this by asking mother a question.

In investigations for follow up evaluation, most useful will be an echocardiogram that will confirm anatomy, function and gradients. An ECG to check for rhythm and electrical activity, Left ventricular hypertrophy if any.

You should following this be prepared for discussion as the case is simple and you should have ample time left till the bell rings.

What is expected from the candidate?
- Introduces self to the mother and John and requests verbal consent.
- Makes it known that hand hygiene has been done before touching the patient.
- Keeps the patient at ease and gives simple and easy to understand commands.
- Inspects and comments on observations.
- Comments presence of scars
- Follows logical sequence to cardiac examination
- Notices and comments on absent left brachial pulse
- Auscultates the back and neck
- Picks up normal heart sounds and murmur
- Works through and evaluates different pathologies
- The candidate should be able to correlate the findings and discuss aetiology and management.

NOTE
If you are asked "Can it be anything else?"

Do not take it as a trick—it may be you might be wrong and the examiner is trying to 'help' you reconsider. If you are sure then say you still think the most likely diagnosis is a coarctation or aortic stenosis say so **but** also mention you will consider a differential including ...."

You should then come out with your differential: "Yes it could be and I would like to consider !: Pulmonary stenosis as the murmur is very close to the area and intensity may be difficult to localize accurately". These can be checked with an echocardiogram"

Do not say "No it cannot be anything else" or "it is classic xyz, you are sure".

This attitude, if you are wrong, suggests you are inflexible and once have made up your mind, are not open to other suggestions. This can be disastrous on a ward when you might be looking after an ill child and may not consider a different aetiology even by pointed out by other members of the team.

In this scenario you will have time to score marks with your discussion. Prepare well and 'lead you discussion':

- Current guidelines on bacterial endocarditis prophylaxis. In UK prophylaxis is not recommended.
- Presentation in newborn period: severe pre-ductal coarctation or critical aortic stenosis.
- Presentation a few hours or days later when ductus arteriosus closes precipitating symptoms. Management of duct dependent lesions.
- Medium to long term out come and need for follow up.

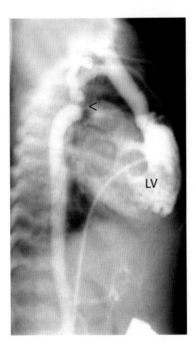

Fig. 21: Angiogram

Left ventricle angiogram showing discrete coarctation of aorta.

On Doppler echocardiogram a high velocity is detected proportional to the degree of obstruction.

CHILD WITH RHEUMATIC HEART DISEASE

Information given to the candidate: You are the candidate and on entering the station, the examiner introduces you to a 12-year-old boy Ram and his mother, both sitting on chair.

Ram has a history of fever when he was 3-year-old and has come for a check as he was noted to have a murmur at the school medical check. He looks well and is in shorts. You are requested to do a cardiovascular examination and any other relevant examination to reach a diagnosis.

You are allowed to talk to the patient but are not allowed to ask any history unless allowed by the examiner.

You have 9 minutes to complete the station; a warning bell will be given at 7 minutes. (UP)

The examination: You introduce yourself to Ram and his mother and obtain a verbal consent. You explain hand hygiene has been adhered to:

On general inspection
• There are no medicine or medical devices around him.
• Ram is 'average size and built'
• He is comfortable, pink, not distressed.
• Chest is normal, normal respiratory rate
• No scars noted

General physical and system exam: Explain to Ram what you will be doing
• No clubbing
• No cyanosis
• Brachial/radial pulse equal, 80/min, regular
• Precordium—no heave or thrill, apex 5th ICS and mid clavicular line
• Heart sounds: 1st and 2nd Normal.
• Holo systolic murmur 2/6, maximal over Mitral area – radiates to axilla
• Does not change with posture
• Femoral pulses are easily palpable

You summarise your findings: You have examined Ram, a 12-year-old boy. He is comfortable at rest. He is pink and seems appropriately grown, but would like to plot him on appropriate chart. There are no scars. He has no clubbing or cyanosis. He has regular pulse, 80/min. Peripheral pulses are easily palpable with no radio-femoral delay. Percordium feels normal with no heaves or thrill. Apex is in midcalvicular line, in 5th ICS. On auscultation his heart sounds 1st and 2nd are heard and are Normal. 2nd is not prominent. *(If you are sure of split sounds—then you can comment on it appropriately or skip it).* there is a systolic murmur grade 2/6, maximal in apex. There are no bruits or murmurs in the neck or the back. You will check his blood pressure

You do not need to stop and can move on to your impression:
In my opinion Ram is well. My most likely differential diagnosis is Mitral regurgitation. I would also like to rule out a VSD. The findings would be suggestive of rheumatic heart disease.

I would like to confirm that by investigations. The most useful will be an echocardiogram that will confirm anatomy and function. An ECG to check for rhythm and electrical activity. If echocardiogram is not available I will also like to do a CXR to look for cardiac size and pulmonary plethora.

You should following this be prepared for discussion as the case is simple and you should have ample time left till the bell rings.

What is expected from the candidate?
- Introduces self to the mother and Ram and requests verbal consent.
- Makes it known that hand hygiene has been done before touching the patient.
- Keeps the patient at ease and gives simple and easy to understand commands.
- Inspects and comments on observations.
- Comments absence of scars
- Follows logical sequence to cardiac examination
- Auscultates the back and neck
- Picks up normal heart sounds and murmur
- Works through and evaluates different pathologies
- The candidate should be able to correlate the findings and discuss aetiology and management.

NOTE

If you are asked "Can it be anything else?"

Do not take it as a trick—it may be you might be wrong and the examiner is trying to 'help' you reconsider. If you are sure then say you still think the most likely diagnosis is a Mitral regurgitation but will consider a differential including ...."

Do *not* be dogmatic in your discussion.

Know rheumatic fever well as examiners may go into discussion on presentation and prophylaxis. Penicillin is recommended till after teenage years.

Rheumatic fever complications are now also seen in the UK and you may encounter this case if taking the exam at an overseas centre.

CYSTIC FIBROSIS

Information given to the candidate

You are the candidate and on entering the station, the examiner introduces you to Anthony, a 12-year-old. He is sitting with his mother.

You are asked to examine his chest and any carry out and other relevant examination to reach a diagnosis.

You are allowed to talk to the patient but are not allowed to ask any history unless allowed by the examiner.

You have 9 minutes to complete the station; a warning bell will be given at 7 minutes. (SP/AG)

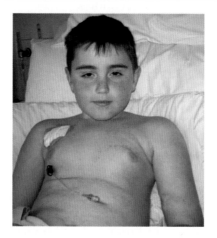

Fig. 22

The examination

You introduce yourself to Anthony and his mother and obtain verbal consent. You explain hand hygiene has been adhered to:

On general inspection
- There are medications on the side table, Creon (Pancreatic enzymes), some antibiotics. There is a Peak flow meter.
- Growth chart with height and weight plotted – on 50th centile. A long line is seen.
- Height and weight appropriate

General physical and system exam
- Clubbing preent
- No cyanosis
- Chest symmetrical
- Equal air entry, no additional sounds
- CVS; Heart sounds: Normal, no murmur.
- Abdomen Soft, liver and spleen not palpable

Confirm that the medicines and the growth chart on the side table are Anthony's.

You summarise your findings: I have examined Anthony, 12-year-old boy. He looks well. On general inspection I note there are some medications on the side table, including Creon. The height and weight are on the 50th centile. Anthony is comfortable at rest and has a long line visible on the right chest wall. There is clubbing, present, but no cyanosis. Chest shape is normal with normal air entry and no additional sounds. Rest of the examination is normal with no hepatosplenomegaly.

You do not need to stop and can move on to your impression:
In my opinion Anthony has cystic fibrosis. He is on regular medication and is very well controlled, evident from his appropriate growth. I would like to check his peak flow.
You should following this be prepared for discussion.

What is expected from the candidate?
- Introduces self to the mother and Anthony and requests verbal consent.
- Makes it known that hand hygiene has been done before touching the patient.
- Keeps the patient at ease and gives simple and easy to understand commands.
- Inspects and comments on observations.
- Works through and concludes differential pathologies
- The candidate should be able to correlate the findings and discuss aetiology and management.

NOTE

On this station there are not many positive clinical findings and hence you should finish quickly. Do not waste time. Be ready for a detailed discussion to score marks.

CYSTIC FIBROSIS

Management

Care for Cystic Fibrosis (CF) is provided by multidisciplinary teams consisting of specialist doctors, nurses, dieticians, physiotherapists and psychologists.

- *Respiratory therapies*
  - Chest physiotherapy: It is very important and should be performed everyday to clear the thick secretions within the lungs. The family members are usually taught how to administer effective physiotherapy.
  - Mucoactive agents are used as an adjunct to physiotherapy to assist in clearing of the secretions. Example: Dornase alpha, hypertonic saline.
  - Antibiotics are given to treat chest infections. They are also used during symptoms of increased cough. They can be given orally, intravenously or nebulised.
  - Antibiotics: For prophylaxis are routinely given by certain centres to decrease the incidence of colonization by *staphylococci*. Flucloxacillin is usually given orally.
  - *Pseudomonas aeruginosa:* It is the current practice to eradicate infections or colonisation with *pseudomonas aeruginosa* whenever it is first isolated. Intravenous, oral and nebulised anti-pseudomonal therapies are given. Most patients require long-term nebulised antibiotics: Colistin, Tobramycin.
  - Azithromycin is also useful in children who are chronically infected with *P. aeruginosa.*
  - Oxygen supplementation at home

- *Gastrointestinal management*
  - It is important to ensure adequate weight gain by providing high calorie diet. A high-fat diet is recommended and further calories can be taken as high energy drinks. In children who may not be able to tolerate the total volume of dietary supplements are fed by an enteral feeding in the short run; but will require a gastrostomy for adequate intake of calories.
  - Pancreatic enzymes are given as required.
  - Vitamin supplements are given specially fat-soluble ones: A, D, E, K
  - Constipation can be a problem and is treated with appropriate laxative.

- *Associated morbidities*
  - Metabolic Bone problems—Osteoporosis and osteopenia are common. Regular monitoring by bone density scans is part of routine management.
  - Liver complications are common and treated with ursodeoxycholic acid. If cirrhosis develops leading to liver failure then liver transplant is considered.
  - Diabetes is managed by insulin and diet control.

Team of specialist doctors should include: Respiratory, endocrine, gastroenterology, hepatic expertise.

Children are seen regularly with yearly evaluation of bloods, lung function and metabolic profile.

- **New therapies**
  - New mucoactive agents
  - Therapies targeting basic effects of CFTR protein function.

Prognosis
Median survival of babies born today with CF is 40 years.

Other relevant information
There about 8,000 patients in the UK. Incidence in Asia is not well established is but the disease is now increasingly seen.

CF is caused by mutation of gene responsible for cystic fibrosis transmembrane regulator (CFTR) on chromosome seven. Currently more than 1200 mutations have been indentified in the gene causing disease.

Most common mutation is: ΔF508del, a deletion of phenylalanine at position 508.

Diagnosis
- Gold standard for diagnosing CF is Sweat test with Chloride > 60 mmol/L.
- Faecal elastase in presence of pancreatic insufficiency. 15% of CF patients are pancreatic sufficient.
- DNA analysis
- Neonatal screening—checks for immune-reactive trypsin (IRT).

RESPIRATORY: CHILD WITH EXACERBATION OF ASTHMA

Information given to the candidate

You are the candidate and on entering, the examiner introduces you to Ikram, a 8-year-old boy. Ikram is sitting on a chair wearing shorts but is completely exposed in the upper half of the body. He looks comfortable and there is a spacer and metered dose inhaler device lying on the table.

The examiner explains that Ikram's father is worried about his breathing and frequent coughs. He requests you to do a respiratory examination any other relevant examination to arrive at a diagnosis.

You are allowed to talk to the patient but not allowed to ask any questions about his condition.

You have 9 minutes to complete the station; a warning bell will be given at 7 minutes.

(Please note patients who are stable and recovering from an acute illness such as exacerbation of asthma, pneumonia, etc. may be brought for exam from an inpatient ward) (SP)

The examination

You introduce yourself to Ikram and his father and obtain a verbal consent from the family. You let the family and examiner know that hand hygiene has been observed. You request Ikram to come to the couch and make sure he is comfortable.

- You look around the room and notice a MDI and spacer lying on the table. He has name bands attached on both his wrists and realise that he is an inpatient.

Explain to Ikram what you will be doing as you go along. On general examination you note:

- He appears tachypneic
- Respiratory rate is 28/min.
- Pulse rate 104/min
- No clubbing
- No pallor or cyanosis (tip of tongue)
- No recessions or scars but minimal tracheal tug.
- Antero-posterior diameter of the chest wall not increased.
- Apex beat is on the left 5th inter-costal space.
- Expansion is equal and symmetrical at the front and back.

You then proceed to percuss the chest wall but the examiner ask you to auscultate:

- Few scattered wheeze and increase in the duration of the expiratory phase on the back

You are then provided with a Wright's peak flow meter by the examiner and informs you that Ikram's height is 122 cm.

- You explain to Ikram how to do a PEFR which he performs with some difficulty and the best score you find is 140 L (3 attempts)
- *You are requested to summarise your findings:* I have examined Ikram, 8-year-old boy. He is mildly tachypneic and not cyanosed and has no clubbing. His chest is symmetrical and seems hyper inflated, i.e. as if in inspiration. He has a wheeze and scattered ronchii on both sides. His PEFR is reduced and I would like to plot it on an appropriate chart. There is a spacer and MDI on the side table. In your opinion Ikram is likely to be recovering from an acute exacerbation of asthma and is probably an inpatient in the ward suggested by the name bands in his wrists.

The ensuing discussion with the examiner is highlighted in the next section.

What is expected from the candidate?
- Introduces self to the father and Ikram and requests verbal consent.
- Makes it known that hand hygiene has been done before touching the patient.
- Alert to note medical devices present near the patient. Enquires whether Ikram is well.
- Keeps the patient at ease and gives simple and easy to understand commands.
- Counts respiratory rate for full 30 seconds with a watch when requested.
- Examines patient on the couch.
- Kneels or sits down by the side of the couch and do not stoop over the patient.
- Comments about the apex beat, chest expansion, respiratory distress and auscultatory findings.
- Candidate is able to demonstrate how to perform PEFR to Ikram. It is not expected of you to remember the normal range—can ask for appropriate data sheet.
- The candidate should be able to correlate the findings of an inpatient (from the wrist bands), tachypneic, mild respiratory distress, wheeze and low PEFR to a child recovering from an acute exacerbation of asthma.

GENERAL NOTE

The discussion about asthma in childhood may include:
1. Investigations for acute asthma being saturation monitoring, PEFR pre- and post-bronchodilator therapy and a CXR to rule an infective cause for the exacerbation.

2. Long term management should include a preventer, checking inhaler technique, paediatrician and an asthma nurse specialist.

3. The PEFR can be performed by a child older than 5 years of age on correct demonstration of the technique, As a rough guidance for a height of 110 cm expected PEFR will be 150 and then for every 10 cm increase in height the PEFR increases by 50 mm, i.e. for a 120 cm tall child PEFR is 200, 130 cm tall child it is 250 and so on (*Source* APLS manual, 4th edition).

4. How to step up and step down treatment in a child with asthma? It is essential for you to know the latest guidelines on asthma, please refer to BTS 2011 guidelines on asthma.

5. A quick way to determine how well controlled the asthma is in a child may be assessed by asking the following questions:
   - Can you run as fast as your friends?
   - If there was a race in your class where would you come?
   - What games do you play (if he says something like football, try to find whether he scores goals or saves goals, i.e. goalkeeper)?
   - How is school (how many days he misses school because of being awake in the night with cough).
   - Can he keep pace with his peers in PE and games(does he need to stop earlier).

http://www.brit-thoracic.org.uk/clinical-information/asthma/asthma-guidelines.aspx

NEUROFIBROMATOSIS NF1

Information given to the candidate

You are the candidate and on entering the station, the examiner introduces you to a 7-year-old girl Joanna and her mother, both sitting on chairs.

Joanna has come for her first appointment, having moved from Spain. She looks well and is in shorts.

You are requested to do a general examination and any other relevant examination to reach a diagnosis.

You are allowed to talk to the patient but are not allowed to ask any history unless allowed by the examiner.

You have 9 minutes to complete the station; a warning bell will be given at 7 minutes. (SE/AG)

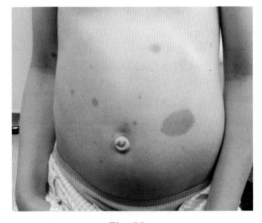

Fig. 23

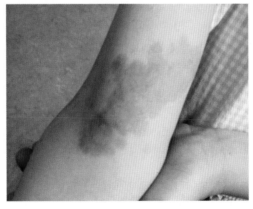

Fig. 24

The examination
You introduce yourself to Joanna and her mother and obtain verbal consent. You explain hand hygiene has been adhered to:

On general inspection
- There are no medications or medical devices around.
- Joanna is 'smallish and of thin built'
- She seems a little 'slow' for her age.
- She is comfortable, pink, not distressed.
- Numerous pigment marks on trunk
- Pigmented lumpy area on her right arm

General physical and system exam
- No clubbing
- No cyanosis
- Pigment macules of different size, 3.0 cm × 2.5 cm biggest
- Raised palpable pigmented lesion right arm
- Freckling in axilla and neck
- Chest—symmetrical, equal movement and air entry
- Precordium—no heave or thrill, apex 5th ICS and mid clavicular line
- Heart sounds: 1st and 2nd Normal. No murmurs.
- Spine is normal

You summarise your findings: You have examined Joanna, a 7-year-old girl. She is comfortable at rest. She is pink and seems small, but would like to plot her on appropriate chart. She has a number of distinct pigmented lesions on trunk. She also has a raised pigmented area on her right arm. There is freckling in the axilla and her neck. She has no clubbing or cyanosis. There are no positive findings in the abdomen—no organomegaly, chest and heart sounds are normal. I would like to check her blood pressure.

You do not need to stop and can move on to your impression: Joanna is well. My findings suggest she is most likely to have neurofibromatosis. I would like to confirm that by genetic testing and get advice from a geneticist. I would also like to have an ophthalmology opinion looking for Lisch nodules.

You should following this be prepared for discussion.

What is expected from the candidate?
- Introduces self to the mother and Joanna and requests verbal consent.
- Makes it known that hand hygiene has been done before touching the patient.
- Keeps the patient at ease and gives simple and easy to understand commands.
- Inspects and comments on observations.
- Comments pigmented areas

- Follows logical sequence to cardiac examination
- Auscultates the back
- Works through and concludes differential pathologies
- The candidate should be able to correlate the findings and discuss aetiology and management.

NOTE

Neurofibromatosis NF1—identified by Friedrich von Recklinghausen. Autosomal dominant.

Management is multidisciplinary with community paediatrician, occupational therapists, teachers and other specialities as needed.

Cognitive
- Lower than average IQ and learning difficulties
- Developmental assessment and support during school years
- ADHD—use CBT and Methylphenidate

Skin
- Café au lait macules are cosmetically distressing but have no effective cure
- Neurofibromas are irritating and painful as they catch on clothes
- Plexiform neurofibromas may turn malignant

Eyes
- Annual ophthalmology check till 7 years of age for risk of optic gliomas.
- Visual acuity checked. A change in acuity requires MRI brain.
- Lisch nodules seen on slit-lamp examination and have no specific treatment

Cardiac
- Check for murmurs – echocardiogram
- Annual BP check
- If hypertensive – check for
  - Renal artery stenosis
  - Pheochromocytoma

Prognosis
Significant morbidity and shortened life expectancy.

Diagnosis
Diagnosis of NF1 is clinical and includes:
- Café au lait macules
  - Six or more. Size 1–3 cm.
  - Benign, hyperpigmented
  - May be present from birth or more prominent in first 2 years
- Freckling of axilla

- Neurofibromas
  - Develop in teens or early 20s.
- Lisch nodules
  - Lesions in iris develop between 5 and 10 years
- Skeletal lesions
  - Short stature
  - Scoliosis
  - Bowing of long bones
- Other clinical features
  - Lower than average IQ
  - Problem with working memory
  - Autistic spectrum disorders
  - Congenital heart defects
  - Renal artery stenosis
  - Malignancies
    - Pheochromocytoma
    - Sarcoma
    - Leukemia
    - GI stromal tumors

Genetics

Due to mutation of NF1 gene on chromosome 17. NF1 gene codes for protein—neurofibromin which acts as a tumour suppressor in the nervous system.

Mutations lead to development of benign and malignant tumors in peripheral nerves and cranial nerve sheaths.

Birth incidence is 1:2500–3000.

CHILD WITH DEXTROCARDIA

Information given to the candidate

You are the candidate and on entering the station, the examiner introduces you to a 12-year-old boy Liam and his father. Liam is lying semi-reclined on the couch wearing shorts but is completely exposed in the upper half of the body. He looks well and sitting comfortably.

The examiner asks you to listen to his chest and do any other relevant examination to arrive at a diagnosis.

You are allowed to talk to the patient but not allowed to ask any questions about his condition.

You have 9 minutes to complete the station; a warning bell will be given at 7 minutes. (SP)

The examination

You introduce yourself to Liam and his father and obtain a verbal consent. You explain hand hygiene has been adhered to:

On general inspection
- There are no medicine or medical devices around him.
- Liam is 'average size and built'
- He is comfortable, pink, not distressed.
- Chest is normal, normal respiratory rate
- No scars noted

General physical and system exam: Explain to Ram what you will be doing
- No clubbing
- No cyanosis
- Brachial/radial pulse equal, 80/min, regular
- Precordium—no heave or thrill, apex difficult to localize in usual position
- Heart sounds: 1st and 2nd are very soft and muffled
- No murmur noted
- Femoral pulses are easily palpable
- You feel heart sounds are better heard on right side
- Difficult to localize apex
- Liver right side—normal location

You summarise your findings: You have examined Liam, a 12-year-old boy. He is comfortable at rest. He is pink and seems appropriately grown, but would like to plot him on appropriate chart. There are no scars. He has no clubbing or cyanosis. He has regular pulse, 80/min. Peripheral pulses are easily palpable with no radio-femoral delay. Precordium feels normal with no heaves or thrill. Apex is difficult to be absolutely sure of. Heart sounds are soft, faint and seem louder on Right side of sternum instead of left. There is no murmur. There are no bruits or murmurs in the neck or the back. Liver is palpable on the right side. I would like to check his blood pressure

You do not need to stop and can move on to your impression:

In my opinion Liam is well. My most likely diagnosis is Dextrocardia. Isolated dextrocardia.

I would like to confirm that by a CXR if needed.

What is expected from the candidate?
• Introduces self to the father and Liam and requests verbal consent.
• Makes it known that hand hygiene has been done before touching the patient.
• Enquires whether Liam is well.
• Keeps the patient at ease and gives simple and easy to understand commands.
• Has examined for clubbing and counted the pulse rate.
• Examines patient semi-reclined at 45°.
• Feels both side of the chest and decides apex beat is on the right side.
• Reconfirms apex beat is actually on right side during auscultation
• Demonstrates percussion as a clinical method of finding liver dullness to decide about situs inversus.
• Offers to look at the nostrils.
• The candidate should be able to correlate the findings of a well patient with apex beat on the right side, no clinical evidence of situs inversus and absence of clubbing and nasal polyps to a case of isolated dextrocardia.
• The discussion with the candidate.

GENERAL NOTE
Dextrocardia is included at this station as it has appeared in respiratory/other station. It is important to locate the apex beat and auscultate carefully so as *not* to miss this comparatively easy case by concentrating on respiratory/breath sounds only.

1. Dextrocardia occurs in approximately 1 in 12,000 people, and one out of 3 will have association with situs inversus.
2. Investigations to rule out situs inversus may include an X-ray, Ultrasound scan of abdomen or a CT scan.
3. Up to 95% cases of situs inversus has congenital heart defects and 25% associated with Kartagener syndrome.
4. Kartagener syndrome is characterised by a triad of symptoms: situs inversus, chronic *sinusitis*, and *bronchiectasis*.

Depending on the associated pathologies a multi-disciplinary team needs to be involved: Paediatrician, respiratory physician, cardiologist, physiotherapist, children's community nurses, etc.

Musculoskeletal and Others

Examination of the Musculoskeletal System in Children

Children are not just miniature adults. Majority of causes relating to musculo-skeletal system (MSK) are trauma related. However, in face of real pathology, management techniques have to be adapted from practice in adults.

While examining a child follow the following rules:

- Look, feel and move.
- Explain what you would do or would like child to do.
- Always ask the child to show the movements she can do without any pain.
- When you are feeling or moving the joints for the range of movements, keep an eye on facial expression.
- Always ask whether it hurts or is painful.

pGALS (paediatric Gait, Arms, Legs, Spine), which is a simple screening approach to MSK examination in school-aged children and may be successfully performed in younger ambulant children.

It is a systematic approach developed in Newcastle and now widely practiced. (http://www.bapn.org/assets/membership)

pGALS—approach to a child presenting with a MSK related symptom will be:

Screening questions may be asked at start or the end of the examination encounter—depending on the task set.

- Do you have any pain or stiffness in your joints, muscles or your back?
- Do you have any difficulty getting yourself dressed without any help?
- Do you have any difficulty going up and down stairs?

GAIT
- Observe the child walking
- Walk on your tip-toes
- Walk on your heels

ARMS
- "Put your hands out in front of you"
- "Turn your hands over and make a fist"
- "Pinch your index finger and thumb together"
- "Touch the tips of your fingers with your thumb"
- Squeeze the metacarpophalangeal joints
- "Put your hands together/put your hands back to back"
- "Reach up and touch the sky"
- "Look at the ceiling"
- "Put your hands behind your neck"

LEGS
- Feel for effusion at the knee
- "Bend and then straighten your knee" (Active movement of knees and examiner feels for crepitus)
- Passive flexion (90 degrees) with internal rotation of hip.

SPINE
- "Open your mouth and put 3 of your (*child's own*) fingers in your mouth"
- Lateral flexion of cervical spine—"Try and touch your shoulder with your ear"
- Observe the spine from behind
- "Can you bend and touch your toes?" Observe curve of the spine from side and behind

We suggest you look up the website for full details. http://www.arthritisresearchuk.org/

For further information about the validation of pGALS see: Foster HE, Kay LJ, Friswell M, Coady D, Myers A. Musculoskeletal screening examination (pGALS) for school-age children based on the adult GALS screen. Arthritis Care Research 2006; 55(5); 709–716.

CHILD WITH RICKETS—VITAMIN-D RESISTANT

Information given to the candidate: You are the candidate and on entering the station, the examiner introduces you to Claire, 6-year-old girl and her mother, both are sitting. Claire looks well and is in shorts. Claire's mother is worried that Claire finds it difficult to run and becomes wobbly.

You are requested to examine musculoskeletal system to reach a diagnosis:

You are allowed to talk to the patient but are not allowed to ask any history unless allowed by the examiner.

You have 9 minutes to complete the station; a warning bell will be given at 7 minutes (SP)

The examination

You introduce yourself to Claire and her mother and obtain a verbal consent from the family.

You notice she looks well and is well grown. You notice she has dental braces and comment on this observation.

You enquire if she has any difficulty in mobilising, climbing stairs and in putting on clothes. Claire replies she needs some help with dressing and finds it difficult to climb stairs.

You request Claire to stand and observe:
• She has bowing of legs with knees wide apart as she is standing with ankles and feet together
• Some muscle wasting in both legs.
• She walks with a waddling gait and a limp.
• Right leg is shortened (coxa vara deformity of hip) leading to the limp

You then go on to examine the hands and observe:
• Mild deformity
• On putting her hands together there is some gap
• Some restriction of movements of the joints due to the deformities
• You ask Claire to insert 3 of her middle fingers into her open mouth and observe
• There is no restriction of the temporomandibular joint.

The examiner then ask you to summarise your findings and give a diagnosis.

You summarise your findings: Claire displays a waddling gait, bow legs (genu varum) and possible deformity of the hip joint (coxa vara deformity). There is some deformity of the upper limbs as she cannot bring her hands together normally. She is wearing dental braces. There is no restriction of her temporomandibular joint.

Claira has evidence of rickets/myopathy. Being a girl and having signs of rickets, Claire may have vitamin-D resistant rickets. The ensuing discussion with the examiner is highlighted in the next section.

What is expected from the candidate?

- Introduces self to the mother and Claire and requests verbal consent.
- Makes it known that hand hygiene has been done before touching the patient.
- Enquires whether Claire can do activities of daily living with ease or needs some help so as to **modify the examination technique without causing pain.**
- Keeps the patient at ease and gives simple, easy to understand instructions.· Inspects gait and comments on bow legs (genu varum) deformity.
- Picks up the waddling gait and suggest hip deformity (coxa vara deformity).
- Explains the myopathy is likely to be due to rickets.
- The candidate should be able to correlate the findings to a myopathy / rickets.
- Being a female patient with signs of rickets, vitamin-D resistant rickets is a likely diagnosis. This is also known as hypophosphatemic rickets.
- **Vit D deficiency is being noted in general population because of limited exposure to sun light and use of sun light blocking creams.**

GENERAL NOTE

This particular case I saw in my examination but does not mean every child with rickets would necessarily be Vit D resistant.

Rickets affects bone development in children. It causes softening and weakening of bones, which can lead to deformities, such as bowed legs and curvature of the spine. This can cause bone tenderness or pain.

The most common cause of rickets is a lack of vitamin D or calcium in the diet. Children from Asian, Afro-Caribbean and Middle Eastern origin are at higher risk because the darker skin needs more sunlight to get enough vitamin D.

Other cause of rickets includes low phosphate as in the case vitamin-D resistant rickets.

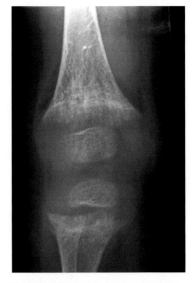

Fig. 25: There is gross expansion of the long bone metaphyses, widening of the growth plate and thinning of the cortices. This appearances are typical of rickets

The discussion about the **vitamin-D resistant rickets** may include:

1. Blood investigations for vitamin-D resistant rickets will show hypophosphataemia, relative normocalcaemia, and normal or low levels of calcitriol
2. Often presents with postnatal growth retardation and dental anomalies. Genu varum (bow legs) deformity will evolve.
3. Has X-linked dominant inheritance pattern and affects about 1 in 20,000 children. Females are more commonly seen with this condition but males may also be found with this condition.
4. Genetic testing will involve checking the alteration in the *PHEX*, i.e. phosphate linked endopeptidase homolog, X-linked gene (Xp22.1).
5. Treatment: Oral phosphate and large doses of vitamin D. Vitamin D therapy in isolation is ineffective
6. Supporting care that may be necessary: Help with mobility, support for parents, genetic counseling for future pregnancies, disability living allowance, physiotherapist, paediatrician, etc.

Coxa vara is a *deformity* of the hip, whereby the angle between the ball and the shaft of the *femur* is reduced to less than 120 degrees. This results in the leg being shortened, and therefore a *limp* occurs. It is commonly caused by injury, such as a fracture. It can also occur when the *bone tissue* in the neck of the *femur* is softer than normal, meaning it bends under the weight of the body.

Ref: http://en.wikipedia.org/wiki/Coxa_vara

OTHER STATION—JUVENILE IDIOPATHIC ARTHRITIS

Information given to the candidate

You are the candidate and on entering the examiner introduces you to Gracie, a 13-year-old girl and her mother. Gracie finds it difficult to keep up with her written assignments.

You are asked to examine Gracie's upper limbs (hands and arms) and any other relevant examination to reach a diagnosis.

You are allowed to talk to the patient but are not allowed to ask any history unless allowed by the examiner.

You have 9 minutes to complete the station; a warning bell will be given at 7 minutes (SE).

The examination

You introduce yourself to Gracie and her mother and obtain a verbal consent from Gracie to examine her.

You note:
- Her hands and feet are swollen and deformed.
- Look around for other clues, i.e. wheelchair, splints, bandages.
- Comment on nutrition (you would like to plot the child's weight and height on charts appropriate for her age and sex.)
- Portacath on left chest wall.

Be sensitive to child / young person's feelings when describing 'abnormal findings in their presence'

Start examination from head to toe by **following pGALS:**
- *Start with neck:* Look up, Put your chin on the chest, touch your ear on your shoulder
- *Temporomandibular joint:* Ask the child to open his mouth and then ask the child to insert three fingers into her mouth
- *Shoulder, Elbow, wrist:* Look for swelling, effusion, warmth, redness and feel for range of movements.
- *Metacarpophalangeal joints and interphalangeal joints:* Ask Gracie to make a fist. Look for the swelling, deformity.
- Ask to demonstrate self help skills like combing the hair, using pencil skills and dressing skills.

Spine: Look for scoliosis.

Gait: Ask whether she is able to walk. If she is able then look for limp and asymmetry of lower limbs. If she is not able to walk, then you may ask whether school has facilities for her wheel chair.

Lower limbs
- Hip, knee and ankle joint: Look for swelling, redness, Feel for effusion. Range of movements
- Look for contractures and scars of contracture release surgeries especially at Achilles tendon. Look for muscle atrophy adjacent to the joints.

She has a portacath in situ for medications.

Look for
- Lymphadenopathy
- Hepatosplenomegaly
- Offer slit-lamp examination to look for uveitis.

Always mention positive findings first and significant negative findings with diagnosis.

Summaries your findings
Gracie is 13-year-old girl with symmetrical swelling of her wrists, knees and ankles. The joints are swollen, not warm or tender. Her metacarpophalangeal and interphalangeal joints are deformed and have restricted movements. There is no lymphadenopathy or hepatosplenomegaly. There is a portacath in situ. Her examination findings suggest that she has juvenile idiopathic arthritis and is needing possibly parenteral medications (methotrexate) in view of port-a-cath. I would like to plot her weight and height on appropriate charts and refer for slit-lamp examination.

What is expected from the candidate?
- Introduces self to Gracie and mother.
- Makes it known that hand hygiene has been done before touching the patient.
- Keeps the patient at ease and gives simple and easy to understand commands.
- Inspects gait and spine and comments on that
- Fluent examination starting from head to toe
- Examines each joint—look, feel and move
- Asks the child whether she is in pain during the examination
- Asks about self help skills and how she manages at school
- Looks for scars, port-a-cath
- Looks for lymphadenopathy and hepatosplenomegaly.
- The candidate should be able to come with the findings and diagnosis.
- The candidate should know the treatment for Juvenile idiopathic arthritis and involvement of multidisciplinary team of physiotherapist, occupational therapist, chiropodists, orthotics and sometimes surgeons.

The examination should be adapted as per pGALS technique. Practice the technique advised so as to be able to do it fluently in the examination.

The discussion will be on, classification, management eg drugs and multidisciplinary team. The limitations in the activities of daily living make this condition as a 'Disability'. Patients are given extra support and disability living allowance etc. in UK. This may be relevant in your discussion and apply this to your local conditions overseas.

The condition can also be present as a history and management station where all of the above would be relevant. You will not need to examine the patient but by questioning should be able to workout limitations to the child's daily living.

Juvenile idiopathic arthritis: Nelson Textbook of Pediatrics.
http://emedicine.medscape.com/article/1007276
http://www.noc.nhs.uk/oxparc/information/diagnoses/a-z/jia.aspx

OTHER EXAMINATION—PROSTHETIC EYE

Information given to the candidate

You are a candidate and on entering the examiner introduces you to William, 8-year-old boy and his mother Ms Casey.

You are requested to examine William's eyes.

William looks well. He is sitting in a chair. His mother is along with him.

You are allowed to talk to the patient but not allowed to take any history from him, unless specified by the examiner.

You have 9 minutes. There will be a warning bell at 7 min (UP).

Examination

Introduce yourself to William and take the opportunity to look around.
General examination: He is well grown. No pallor, jaundice.

- Look for spontaneous eye movement, nystagmus, coloboma, telengiectasia, colour of the iris, etc.

Testing vision
- Ask him to read the days on a calendar/picture on the wall.
- Ask him to cover one eye individually and read the number again.

You find out that he cannot see with his right eye.

Test for range of eye movements, field of vision.
- Normal range of movement – even on right eye
- No vision in right eye

Seek permission to shine bight light into each eye.
- Check for direct and consensual light reflex.
- Absent light reflex in right eye.
- Offer to do fundoscopy

You may well ask for palpating the eyeballs and can appreciate that right eyeball more harder than left one.

Summarize your finding:

William 8-year-old looks well and comfortable. His right eye does not have any vision and does not respond to light reflex. Fundoscopy examination reveal no light reflex in right eye. Right eye feels harder than left.

I think William has a prosthetic right eye. The cause is likely to be due to retinoblastoma, congenital blindness, congenital glaucoma, etc.

What is expected from the candidate?
- Introduce yourself to William and seek verbal consent.
- Follow hand hygiene
- Keep the patient comfortable and try to build a rapport.
- Identify the absent vision in right eye.
- Able to do sleek ophthalmological examination.
- To seek permission for fundoscopy examination and should be able to give clear and simple instruction to the patient.
- Able to discuss the differentials.
- Supporting care in form of DLA, child psychiatry, educational support, support for parents may need to be discussed as well.

Differential diagnosis of blindness—unilateral in children.

GOITRE

Information given to the candidate

You are the candidate and on entering, the examiner introduces you to Sophie 14-year-old girl and her mother. Sophie was referred by GP for not doing well at school and being lethargic.

You are asked to examine her neck and any further relevant system to reach a diagnosis

You are allowed to talk to the patient but are not allowed to ask any history unless allowed by the examiner.

You have 9 minutes to complete the station; a warning bell will be given at 7 minutes (SE)

Examination

You introduce yourself to Sophie and her mother and obtain a verbal consent from Sophie to examine her.

You notice
- A swelling in her neck .
- General nutritional status (plot the child's weight and height on charts appropriate for her age and sex)
- Whether she looks flushed or anxious.
- Voice for hoarseness

Start with examination of the neck swelling from the front.

Inspection
- Swelling is uniform or unilateral nodular.
- Any scars.
- To drink water from a glass and confirm that the swelling moves up with swallowing.
- Stick out tongue – swelling should not rise with the manoeuvre.
- Eyes: exophthalmos – comment if Normal

Palpation
- Always palpate the swelling from behind the child.
- Inform the child of how you will examine and be Gentle.
- Estimate the size, mention shape and surface constituency.
- Try and get below the swelling.
- Ask the child to drink while you are palpating.
- Check for lymphadenopathy

Look for eye signs from behind—See for exophthalmos from above and behind.

Percuss sternum for retrosternal extension.

Auscultate for bruit.

Proceed to access the thyroid status.

- Eyes: Exophthalmos, eyelid oedema and lid lag
- Hand: Cold/warm, sweaty, fine tremors, clubbing
- Pulse: Tachycardia or bradycardia
- CVS: Hyperactive precordium
- CNS: Delayed reflexes relaxation and proximal muscle weakness.
  Mention that you would like assess her pubertal status.

Summarize

Sophie is 14-year-old girl with a smooth goitre. She has no signs of hypothyroidism or thyrotoxicosis. She may be well controlled on medications or it is a pubertal goitre.

What is expected from the candidate?

- Introduces self to Sophie and mother.
- Makes it known that hand hygiene has been done before touching the patient.
- Keeps the patient at ease and gives simple and easy to understand commands.
- Fluent examination starting from front and back.
- Swelling-inspection, palpation, percussion and auscultation.
- Looks for eye signs from behind: Looks for the signs of thyroid status.
- The candidate should be able to come with the findings and diagnosis.
- The candidate should know the investigations and treatment for goitre.

Thyroid involvement is common in pubertal girls as presenting with enlarged gland.

It can also be a part of multi-gland involvement that affects: Thyroid, adrenals and the ovaries.

Polyglandular autoimmune (PGA) syndromes (otherwise known as polyglandular failure syndromes) are constellations of multiple endocrine gland insufficiencies.

Differential of midline swelling in neck:
- Thyroid swelling
- Thyroglossal cyst
- Cystic hygroma

http://emedicine.medscape.com/article/124183-overview

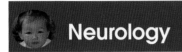

CHILD WITH HEMIPLEGIA

Information given to the candidate

You are the candidate and on entering the station, the examiner introduces you to a 7-year-old boy Aaron and his mother, both are sitting on chairs. You are requested to do a neurological examination of his lower limbs and any other relevant examination to reach a diagnosis. You are allowed to talk to the patient but are not allowed to ask any history unless allowed by the examiner.

Aaron looks well and is wearing shorts.

You have 9 minutes to complete the station; a warning bell will be given at 7 minutes. (SP)

The examination

You introduce yourself to Aaron and his mother and obtain a verbal consent from the family. You notice he is well, wearing spectacles and his head looks relatively big for his stature.

You request Aaron to stand and notice:
• Limb length discrepancy with left lower limb shorter than the right
• Muscle atrophy on the left.

On walking
• He walks with a swinging motion in a semi-circular way of his leg
• His left arm is semi-flexed which becomes more apparent when he runs.

You examine his back
• There are no deformities or scar. You let the examiner know you findings.

You ask Aaron to come to the couch and lie down.
• Reconfirm the finding of apparent limb length discrepancy.
• Notice scars on the left ankle which you inform the examiner, are likely to be due to tendon release operation.
• On moving his lower limbs, some restriction on the left side.
• On passive movements there is increased tone in the left side
• Clonus in his left ankle joint.
• Reduced power on the left lower limb—it is 4/5 in MRC scale.
• Reflexes—notice that the plantar is up going on the left side
• Exaggerated reflexes on the left knee and ankle joints.

You say that you want to examine the upper limbs but the examiner stops you and says that you will find similar findings in the upper limb as well.

The examiner asks you to summarise your findings.

You summarise your findings: I have examined Aaron, a 7-year-old boy. He displays a hemiplegic gait with left lower limb wasting, hypertonic muscles, up going planters, clonus and exaggerated reflexes which will fit in with a upper motor neurone lesion. He has scar on his left ankle which may be due to tendon release operation.

The examiner then shows you a small scar on the right upper part of the abdomen and asks you to comment on that and its relevance to your clinical findings. You take a pause and gather your thoughts on the clinical scenario. Your initial observation suddenly flashes in your mind and you ask Aaron whether it is fine to feel his head. Aaron is happy about that and on feeling the head you feel a button like elevated object at the side of his head.

The button like structure in the head is likely the reservoir of a ventricular shunt which also accounts for the abdominal scar. In essence Aaron has hydrocephalus which will explain the findings demonstrated. It may be related to Aaron being premature and suffering and cerebral haemorrhage (intraventricular haemorrhage) leading to hydrocephalus and hemiplegia.

Further discussion should be on management.

What is expected from the candidate?
- Introduces self to the mother and Aaron and requests verbal consent.
- Makes it known that hand hygiene has been done before touching the patient.
- Keeps the patient at ease and gives simple and easy to understand commands.
- Inspects gait and comments on that.
- Picks up the hemiplegic gait along with the upper limb semi-flexed posture while running.
- Inspects the back and also comments on the scars in ankle
- Comments on left limb spasticity and clonus
- Demonstrates exaggerated reflexes
- When the abdominal scar is shown the candidate should consider examining the head to actively look for the hydrocephalus reservoir.
- The candidate should be able to correlate the findings of an upper motor neurone lesion, the reservoir and abdominal scar as a consequence of hydrocephalus which will explain a unifying diagnosis.

NOTE

- **Supporting care that may be necessary: Help with mobility, support for parents, disability living allowance, physiotherapist, community paediatrician supervision.**
- Premature children are followed by Community Paediatricians for their development in a multidisciplinary setting. The aim is to detect any abnormalities early and provide effective intervention.
- Special schooling is available to the needy children. There is a drive to keep children in main stream schools, with additional help, as far as possible.

CHILD WITH DUCHENNE'S MUSCULAR DYSTROPHY

Information given to the candidate

You are the candidate and on entering the station, the examiner introduces you to an 8-year-old boy Iqbal and his mother, both sitting. You are requested to do a neurological examination of his lower limbs and any other relevant examination to reach a diagnosis. You are allowed to talk to the patient but are not allowed to ask any history unless allowed by the examiner.

Iqbal looks well and is in shorts.

You have 9 minutes to complete the station; a warning bell will be given at 7 minutes. (SP)

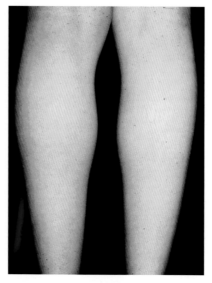

Fig. 26

The examination

You introduce yourself to Iqbal and his mother and obtain a verbal consent from the family.

You notice he looks well and is well grown.

You request Iqbal to stand:
- Notice his calf muscles on both sides looks hypertrophied in comparison to the thigh muscles.
- On walking there is a waddling gait.
- On running he falls on the floor and is upset.

You offer an apology to Iqbal and ask him whether he is hurt to which he confirms he is not.

• You observe him trying to stand up and in the process notice Gower's sign.

   The examiner asks you to elicit the reflexes. You explain to Iqbal that you are going to make his legs jump with this rubber hammer and allow him to feel the hammer before checking the reflexes.

• Knee jerk normal and are not brisk.

• Ankle reflex cannot be elicited

• You try to elicit it again by asking Iqbal to close his eyes and pull his fingers like a hook when you request him to do so (Jendrassik manoeuvre) but are still unable to elicit ankle jerk.

You thank Iqbal and request him to take a seat.

There is a knock on the door.

You turn to the examiner to summarize your findings:
You summarise your findings: I have examined Iqbal, an 8 years old boy. He looks well and comfortable. He has hypertrophy of the calf muscles and on walking has a waddling gait. He has muscle weakness as when he stood up following a fall, he demonstrated 'Gower's sign'. His muscle tone feels normal, knee jerks can be elicited but I could not elicit ankle reflexes even with reinforcement.

You need not stop and continue: Putting the findings together Duchenne's muscular dystrophy is the likely diagnosis.

The discussion with the examiner is highlighted in the next section.

What is expected from the candidate?
Introduces self to the mother and Iqbal and requests verbal consent.

Makes it known that hand hygiene has been done before touching the patient.

Keeps the patient at ease and gives simple and easy to understand commands.

Inspects gait and comments on that.

Picks up the waddling gait and calf muscle hypertrophy.

When the child falls offers an apology and makes sure that the child is not hurt.

Observes and comments on the Gower's sign while Iqbal tries to stand.

Demonstrates reflexes and applies reinforcement technique before concluding that ankle reflexes are absent.

The candidate should be able to correlate the findings of a male patient, calf muscle hypertrophy, positive Gower's sign and absent ankle reflexes with Duchenne's muscular dystrophy as a unifying diagnosis.

The discussion with the candidate may include:
1. Blood investigations for Duchenne's muscular dystrophy being raised Creatinine kinase (CK) and raised AST.
2. Often presents with delayed walking
3. Has X-linked recessive inheritance pattern and affects about 1 in 4,000 males, some females may show mild symptoms. Life limiting condition.
4. Genetic testing will involve checking the mutation in the dystrophin gene, located in humans on the X chromosome (Xp21).
5. Supporting care that may be necessary: Help with mobility, support for parents, genetic counseling for future pregnancies, disability living allowance, physiotherapist, community paediatrician supervision.

The examiner is unlikely to ask you so early in the station to elicit the reflexes in most cases. You should do it yourself.

TUBEROUS SCLEROSIS COMPLEX

Information given to the candidate

You are the candidate and on entering the station, the examiner introduces you to Tilak is a 9-year-old. He has come to the out patients clinic for a follow up. He is sitting with his father.

Please perform relevant examination and arrive at a provisional diagnosis.

You are allowed to talk to the patient but are not allowed to ask any history unless allowed by the examiner.

You have 9 minutes to complete the station; a warning bell will be given at 7 minutes. (AG)

The examination

You introduce yourself to Tilak and his mother and obtain verbal consent

• You explain hand hygiene has been adhered to

On general inspection

• There are no medications or medical devices around.
• Acneiform rash on the cheeks.

General physical and system exam: Adequate exposure is important

• No clubbing
• No cyanosis
• Acneiform rash on cheeks (Adenoma Sebaceum—facial skin hamartomas)
• Hypopigmented areas on the back(Ash leaf macules)
• Leathery, irregular area over lumbar region (Shagreen patch)
• Café au lait spots

Examiner offers you opportunity to ask 2 questions:

You ask:

• *Is Tilak on any medications?*: Yes, he is on Epilim (Sodium Valproate) twice a day (anti-epileptic medications).
• *Which school does he go to?* He has learning difficulties and but goes to a local school.

You summarise your findings:

Tilak is a 9-year-old boy who has adenoma sebaceum, ash leaf macules and café au lait spots on his arms and trunks. He also has an irregular, fibrous area on his lumbar region.

I would like to complete my examination by plotting his weight and height on a growth chart and recording his blood pressure. I would also like to do a full developmental assessment.

You do not need to stop and can move on to your impression:

In addition as Tilak is on anti-epileptic medications and has learning difficulties it is likely that he has tuberous sclerosis.

You should following this be prepared for discussion.

The examiner asks if any clinical aid would help you with your diagnosis in an outpatient set-up.

You answer that a UV or Wood's light would help to demonstrate the ash leaf macules more clearly.

The examiner then asks if there are any other systems you would like to examine.

You reply that ideally you would like to perform a fundoscopy to look for retinal hamartomas and do a cardiovascular examination, requesting an echocardiogram as rhabdomyomas may be associated with this condition and cannot be detected clinically.

What is expected from the candidate?
- Introduces self to the mother and requests verbal consent.
- Makes it known that hand hygiene has been done before touching the patient.
- Keeps the patient at ease and gives simple and easy to understand commands.
- Inspects and comments on observations.
- Works through and concludes differential pathologies
- The candidate should be able to correlate the findings and discuss aetiology and management.

NOTE

Tuberous sclerosis is a autosomal dominantly inherited condition.

Patients have deletions on chromosome 9 (TSC1 gene) or Chromosome 16 (TSC2 gene). Mutations in the hamartin gene account for approximately half of the cases (TSC1) and the other half arise due to mutations in the tuberin gene (TSC2).

Features

Dermatologic
- Adenoma sebaceum is an angiofibroma (cutaneous hamartoma)—usually occurs in late childhood/early adolescence. Initially appears as flat reddish macular lesions. Papular nodules can be seen over the cheeks and bridge of the nose.
- Ash leaf macules: Hypomelanotic patches

- Shagreen patch: Thickened area of connective tissue on the lower back
- Periungual fibroma: Outgrowth from nail beds which usually do not appear until puberty
- Café au lait spots are seen occasionally.

Neurologic
- Seizures are most common presenting symptom and will occur in 90% of young people. Infantile spasms occur in one-third.
- MRI shows tubers, subependymal nodules or subependymal giant cell astrocytomas. CT is less sensitive and subependymal calcification may not occur until the 2nd year of life.

Learning difficulties
- Occurs in up to 40–50% of children with TSC. There is a strong association between TSC and autism particularly as an outcome of infantile spasms.

Cardiac
- Rhabdomyomas of the heart may be asymptomatic but can lead to outflow obstruction, conduction difficulties and death.

Renal
- Renal cysts and angiomyolipomas are noted in 45–50% of people with TCS.

Eye
- Retinal hamartomas.

Management
- MDT approach involving paediatrician, neurologist, cardiologist, nephrologist, ophthalmologist, community team and geneticist.
- Seizure control and management of behavioural problems
- Assessment of learning difficulties as these children may need extra support Genetic counselling and family screening to be offered to families.

CHILD WITH BENIGN ESSENTIAL TREMOR

Information given to the candidate

You are the candidate and on entering the station, the examiner introduces you to Lauren, 15-year-old girl and her mother, both sitting. Lauren looks well and comfortable. The examiner explains Lauren has come for a review as she is having problems and finds it particularly difficult to brush her hair, writing at school and using cutleries.

You are requested to examine her hands and any other relevant examination to reach a diagnosis

You are allowed to talk to the patient to ask a few relevant questions regarding her symptoms unless stopped by the examiner. You are not expected to ask any personal questions.

You have 9 minutes to complete the station; a warning bell will be given at 7 minutes (SP).

The examination

You introduce yourself to Lauren and her mother and obtain a verbal consent from the family. You notice she looks healthy and well grown. You reiterate the history you gathered from the examiner to Lauren and ask her how long she has noticed it as a problem? Lauren replied as long as she can remember. You check how she has been off late with particular **emphasis about any recent sore throat and fever**. Lauren replies there was none. You then ask Lauren about her school to which she says everything is fine. At this point Lauren's mother intervenes that school has picked up the tremor as a problem.

- You then explain to Lauren that you are going to examine her hands and she will have to shake hands, grip your finger and a few other 'tricks'.
- When you offer your hand to Lauren for **handshake**, you notice that she has some tremor while putting her hand forward but the grip is normal, her palms are not sweaty or hot, and relaxes her grip without any delay.
- Lauren **puts her hands forward** and spread her fingers, you put a sheet of paper on top of her hands and demonstrate **tremor**. You then ask her to hold the paper between her fingers and notice that the grip is normal.
- You ask Lauren to write her full name on a piece of paper. You notice this is difficult, there is tremor and she exhibits dysgraphia.
- The finger nose co-ordination test does not reveal past pointing.
- Her **gait** is normal and no abnormality is noted while walking and moving

You ask for permission to examine Lauren to exclude hyperthyroidism.
- No swelling seen in the neck. You then ask Lauren to show her tongue and do not notice any movement in the neck and also her tongue looks normal. You look over her head and do not find any exophthalmos.

- You then request Lauren to follow your finger with her eyes keeping her head still. You do not elicit any lid lag.
- You request the examiner for a glass of water to see movement of thyroid gland. The examiner asks you whether you see any swelling in the neck and you reply there is none. You are advised that it is not necessary to demonstrate the swallowing.

You ask about drug history and Lauren says that she is on a medicine although she is not on oral contraceptive pills.

The examiner then asks you to summarise your findings.

You summarise your findings: I have examined Lauren, 15-year-old girl. She is comfortable and pink. There is no obvious clubbing. The power and tone in her arms is normal. Lauren displays tremor of hands, a normal gait, normal cerebellar signs, and no evidence of myopathy or hyperthyroidism. In your opinion she is likely to have benign essential tremors.

The ensuing discussion with the examiner is highlighted in the next section.

What is expected from the candidate?
- Introduces self to the mother and Lauren and requests verbal consent.·
  Makes it known that hand hygiene has been done before touching the patient.
- Enquires whether Lauren is well and asks relevant questions to decide whether the tremor is a new onset one.
- Keeps the patient at ease and gives simple and easy to understand commands.
- Inspects and comments on grip, gait.
- Goes on to examine for evidence of hyperthyroidism and cerebellar signs but is attentive to comments from the family and examiner.
- Demonstrates tremor causing problem with writing hence face problem at school.
- The candidate should be able to correlate the findings of a well patient and signs of ongoing tremor (Lauren commented she has this problem as long as she can remember) with a benign essential tremor as the likely diagnosis.

GENERAL NOTE

The discussion about the benign essential tremor may include:
1. Benign essential tremor can start in early childhood but gets noted as a problem as the complexities of educational needs increases such as writing, doing work in the laboratory, e.g. handling chemicals, glass test tubes.
2. One of the parents may have this in up to 50% of cases.
3. Treatment: Beta-blockers such as propanolol may be used if hampering activities of daily living such as writing, using cutleries, brushing teeth, etc.
4. Supporting care that may be necessary: Extra time as school to complete tasks such as writing, psychological support if issues with bullying, paediatrician to monitor progress, medicines, etc.

CHILD WITH CONGENITAL MYOTONIC DYSTROPHY

Information given to the candidate

You are the candidate and on entering the examiner introduces you to Ashley, a 4-year-old girl and her mother. The examiner explains that Ashley had problem with breathing in the newborn period and needed feeding support for a period of time. **You are requested to observe and comment on her features and then do the relevant examination to reach a diagnosis.** You are allowed to talk to the patient but are not allowed to ask any history unless allowed by the examiner.

You have 9 minutes to complete the station; a warning bell will be given at 7 minutes. (SP)

The examination

You introduce yourself to Ashley and her mother and obtain a verbal consent. You let the examiner and the mother know that hand hygiene has been observed.

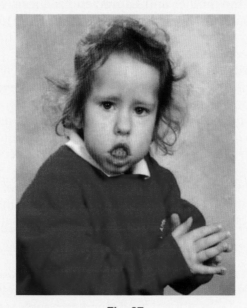

Fig. 27

You note Ashley:
- Is comfortable and happy at rest.
- Is drooling saliva.
- Looks small and would like to plot her parameters on a growth chart.
- Has a long face, small mouth and has got no creases on the forehead.

- Mumbles something which her mother understands and smiles when you try and speak to her.
- Mother took a while to smile at her.

You now want to do a **neurological examination of the lower limbs**.
- You request Ashley to walk and notice she found it difficult to get up from the chair and walk.
- Notice that she is walking with a waddling gait.
- When asked to run she does not manage to do so.
- You also notice that Ashley does not have much muscle mass.
- You then go on to do muscle tone and found it quite easy to do passive movements although you could not elicit the power as Ashley becomes distressed at this stage.

You thank Ashley and request her to take a seat.

There is a knock on the door. The examiner asks you to shake hands with the mother and then summarise your findings.
- *You summarise:* Ashley displays a myotonic facies, waddling gait, muscle atrophy, poor truncal tone, Gastrostomy peg in situ for feeding and absent ankle reflexes even with reinforcement.
- You also say that Ashley's mum was slow releasing the grip while you shook hands with her and that you earlier noticed that she took longer to smile at Ashley than you would expect.
- You say that putting findings together congenital myotonic dystrophy is a likely diagnosis.

The examiner asks you to demonstrate the reflexes.
- You explain to Ashley that you are going to make her legs jump with a rubber hammer and allow her to feel the hammer before checking the reflexes
- With reinforcement you manage to elicit the knee reflexes which you notice being slow
- You are unable to demonstrate the ankle jerks (with reinforcement).
- You then ask Ashley to sit up which she does with some difficulty and delay.
- You now notice a gastrostomy peg in situ and a transverse scar in the upper abdomen.

The discussion with the examiner is highlighted in the next section.

What is expected from the candidate?
- Introduces self to the mother and Ashley and requests verbal consent.
- Makes it known that hand hygiene has been done before touching the patient.
- Keeps the patient at ease and gives simple and easy to understand commands.
- Comment on myotonic facies with empathy and respect.

- Inspects gait and comments on that.
- Picks up the waddling gait and muscle atrophy.
- Observes poor truncal tone when Ashley tries to sit up.
- Demonstrates reflexes and applies reinforcement technique before concluding that ankle reflexes are absent.

The candidate should be able to correlate the findings of a girl who in the newborn period had respiratory and feeding issues, muscle atrophy, poor truncal tone, feeding device in situ, slow releasing grip in mother and absent ankle reflexes with Congenital myotonic dystrophy as a unifying diagnosis.

GENERAL NOTE

The discussion about congenital myotonic dystrophy may include:
1. Blood investigations for congenital myotonic dystrophy being raised Creatinine kinase (CK) and raised AST.
2. Often presents with respiratory and feeding issues in the neonatal period. Can have decreased movement in utero.
3. Has autosomal dominant inheritance pattern and affects males and females.
4. Anticipation phenomenon is demonstrated in congenital myotonic dystrophy. Genetic testing may involve checking the mutation in the **unstable region in the** *DMPK* **gene**.
5. Supporting care that may be necessary:
   - Help with mobility,
   - Disability living allowance,
   - Physiotherapist,
   - Dietitian,
   - Community paediatrician input
   - Support for parents,
   - Genetic counseling for future pregnancies
6. Differential diagnosis:
   - Cerebral palsy,
   - Congenital muscular dystrophy,
   - Limb-Girdle muscular dystrophy,
   - Metabolic myopathies,
   - Myasthenia gravis,
   - Spinal muscular atrophy.

CNS EXAMINATION—GUILLAIN-BARRÉ SYNDROME

Information given to the candidate

You are the candidate and you are introduced to Ravi, 11-year-old boy and his mother. The examiner explains that Ravi has been having difficulty in walking for past few weeks. **Please examine the peripheral nervous system. He is lying on the examination couch.**

You are allowed to talk to the patient but not allowed to take history from him unless specified by the examiner.

You have 9 minutes. There will be a warning bell at 7 min (UP).

Examination

Introduce yourself to Ravi and take the opportunity to look around and you see there is a wheelchair beside the couch.

General examination: He is well grown. No other positive findings

Further examination you note
- Muscle bulk normal no visible atrophy
- Reduced tone in his lower limbs.
- Power is grade 3/5 in ankle, knee and hip joint
- Power in upper arm is grade 5/5.
- Ankle reflex is absent in both lower limb.
- Knee jerks are present.
- Planter responses are flexor.
- Sensory system: No sensory loss.

Offer to examine cranial nerves and spirometry.

Turn to examiner and summarise your finding:

Ravi is 8-year-old looks well and comfortably lying flat. He has decrease tone in lower limb. His tendon reflexes are depressed in lower limb. He has symmetrical loss of power in muscles in the lower limbs I would like to complete my examination with examination of his cranial nerves. My provisional diagnosis is symmetrical lower motor neuron involvement of lower limb most likely due to Guillain-Barré syndrome in the recovery stage.

What is expected from the candidate?
- Introduce yourself to Ravi and seek verbal consent.
- Follow hand hygiene
- Keep the patient comfortable and try to build a rapport.
- Give clear instruction to patient.
- To perform sleek neurology examination.
- To identify lower motor neuron lesion.

- To correlate symmetrical distal paralysis with GBS as a probable diagnosis.
- Should offer to examine cranial nerves.
- Should offer to do spirometry and BP monitoring (commonest complication)
- Able to know the common condition and differential between anterior horn cell, nerves, and muscle involvement.
- Should be aware of the prognostic indicator.
- Supporting care in form of physiotherapy, occupational therapy, DLA, child psychiatry, educational support, support for parents may need to be discussed as well.

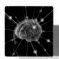

Remember !

Listen to and focus on the task set
Do NOT upset the child
Look for genetic / neuro-cutaneous syndromes and MENTION them

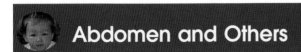

Abdomen and Others

ABDOMEN: CHILD WITH HEREDITARY SPHEROCYTOSIS

Information given to the candidate

You are the candidate and on entering the station, the examiner introduces you to Ashley, a 10-year-old boy and his father. The examiner explains that father is concerned about Ashley looking pale and yellow intermittently. Ashley is lying semi-reclined on the couch wearing shorts but is completely exposed in the upper half of the body. He looks well and comfortable.

You are requested to examine his abdomen and any other system to arrive at a diagnosis

You are allowed to talk to the patient but not allowed to ask any questions about his condition unless allowed by the examiner.

You have 9 minutes to complete the station; a warning bell will be given at 7 minutes (SP)

The examination

You introduce yourself to Ashley and his father and obtain a verbal consent. You note he looks healthy and well grown. You let the family know that hand hygiene has been observed.

You do a quick general examination:
- No clubbing
- Pulse rate 78/min
- Inspect the sclera, it looks yellow (You take Ashley by the window to examine under natural sunlight). Yellow tinge is noted under the tongue.
- Dental hygiene appears good.

Ashley then comes back to the couch and you kneel down for abdominal examination:
- Inspection of the abdominal wall—no scars or abnormality.
- Palpation (explain to Ashley that you are going to feel his tummy gently) and keep your gaze on his face.
- Splenomegaly is found about 5 finger breadth from the inter-costal margin.
- No hepatomegaly.
- Percussion note is tympanitic
- Auscultation reveals normal bowel sounds.
- You should offer to examine the genitalia and anus although the examiner will not let you proceed unless there are some signs to be found.

The examiner then asks you to ask father 2 relevant questions and then summarise your findings. You ask the father whether there is any history of long term jaundice and splenectomies in the family. He replies in the affirmative for both.

You summarise your findings and say that Ashley appears well with evidence of jaundice. There are no scars on the abodmen; the spleen is palpable 5 cm below the costal margin. With a family history of jaundice and splenectomies and being of Caucasian origin you explain that Hereditary spherocytosis is the most likely diagnosis in this case.

The ensuing discussion with the examiner is highlighted in the next section.

What is expected from the candidate?
- Introduces self to the father and Ashley and requests verbal consent.
- Makes it known that hand hygiene has been done before touching the patient.
- Enquires whether Ashley is well.
- Keeps the patient at ease and gives simple and easy to understand commands.
- Has examined for icterus in natural sunlight by taking child to the window for natural sunlight.
- Examines patient lying flat on the couch.
- Kneels down by the side of the couch and do not stoop over the patient.
- Keeps eye on the face to detect any tenderness.
- Provides a realistic measure of the splenomegaly by finger breadths but should be ready to measure it formally if advised by the examiner.
- Demonstrates percussion to find liver dullness and rule out hepatomegaly and completes the station by doing an auscultation.
- The candidate should be able to correlate the findings of a well Caucasian patient with jaundice and splenomegaly to Hereditary spherocytosis.

As you finished the station, the examiner informed you that Ashley's father is on long term folic acid and had a splenectomy 10 years back.

GENERAL NOTE

To add differential diagnosis of a large spleen.

The discussion about hereditary spherocytosis may include:
1. Hereditary spherocytosis is an autosomal dominant condition.
2. Folic acid supplementation and penicillin prophylaxis is necessary.
3. At higher risk of invasive infection from encapsulated organisms such as *Pneumococcus, Meningococcus* and *Haemophilus influenzae*. Suggested repeat booster dose of vaccination every 5 years and before splenectomy.

4. Regular follow-up with a paediatrician and haematologist necessary.
5. Avoidance of contact sports advisable.
6. Regular monitoring of haemoglobin and reticulocyte counts.
7. Genetic counseling for future pregnancies.
8. Another diagnosis to consider in the exam situation is Sickle cell disease (Afro-Caribbean child).

ABDOMINAL /OTHER—BILIARY ATRESIA

Information given to the candidate

You are the candidate and on entering the station, the examiner introduces you to John 5-month-old boy and his mother.

You are requested to do a abdominal examination and any other relevant examination to reach a diagnosis.

You are allowed to talk to the patient and parent but are not allowed to ask any history unless allowed by the examiner.

You have 9 minutes to complete the station; a warning bell will be given at 7 minutes (SE).

Examination

You introduce yourself to John's mother and obtain a verbal consent from mum to examine him. You tell mum that you would like to undress the baby to nappies.

General examination: You notice
- Nutritional status
- Jaundiced—skin as well as sclera is icteric.
- Nasogastric tube in situ
- Hickman line.
- No clubbing, palmer erythema, lyphadenopathy, spider nevi

Abdominal examination
- Mild abdominal distension
- No tenderness
- Small scar in right upper quadrant
- No dilated veins
- 1 cm hepatomegaly which is not tender
- No splenomegaly or
- No free fluid by shifting dullness
- Open the nappy and look for any stools or any urine.
- Nappy has stools.

If there is any stool, comment on the colour, whether it is white coloured stool which will give you a indication of the cause of the jaundice.

Say that you would like to plot the child's weight, height and head circumference on charts appropriate for his age and sex.

Summaries the examination

Always mention positive findings first and significant negative findings with diagnosis.

John is 5-month-old boy with jaundice and hepatomegaly with NG tube and Hickman line with a small scar suggestive of liver biopsy with no signs of chronic liver failure. Most probable diagnosis is biliary atresia. Other possibilities are congenital infections like TORCH and metabolic conditions given the age of the child.

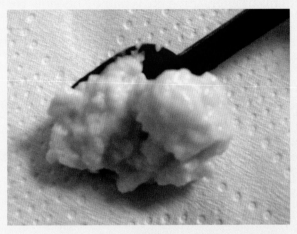

Fig. 28

What is expected from the candidate?
- Introduces self and greets John and his mother.
- Makes it known that hand hygiene has been done before touching the patient.
- Is gentle with the child.
- Undresses the child.
- Fluent examination starting from head to toe
- Looks for scars, notices hickman line.
- Looks for lymphadenopathy and hepatosplenomegaly.
- The candidate should be able to come with the findings and diagnosis.
- The candidate should know the investigations of neonatal jaundice in terms of blood test, ultrasound and liver biopsy.
- Should know the Kasai surgery and timing of the surgery in respect to success rates.

GENERAL NOTE
- Check out biliary atresia, investigations.
- Levels of acceptable total and direct bilirubin levels.

ABDOMEN: CHILD WITH BILIARY ATRESIA STATUS POST KASAI'S PROCEDURE

Information given to the candidate

You are the candidate and on entering the station, the examiner introduces you to a 1-year-old Asian boy John and his mother Ms Baby. John is lying flat on the couch with his mother sitting on a chair by his side. He is only wearing a vest. He looks comfortable.

The examiner asks you to examine the abdominal and discuss possible diagnosis.

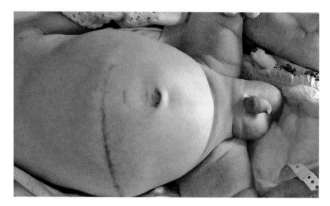

Fig. 29

You are allowed to talk to the mother but not allowed to ask any questions about his condition.

You have 9 minutes to complete the station; a warning bell will be given at 7 minutes (SP/AG)

The examination

You introduce yourself to Ms Baby and obtain a verbal consent from her. You inform that hand hygiene has been observed.

On general inspection
- There are no medications or medical devices around.
- John looks small for his age
- Note has a large scar on the abdomen plus 2 small scars
- Distended abdomen

General physical and system exam: Adequate exposure is important
- Mild jaundice—icteric
- No clubbing

- No cyanosis
- Pulse 120/min
- Back of hands number of whitish marks—star like

Inform you will now feel the abdomen
- Liver—4 cm below coastal margin. Firm, non-tender
- Spleen—3 cm below coastal margin
- Hernial sites—Left inguinal hernia
- Genitalia: Hydrocele right testicle

Request mothers help to elicit fluid thrill and the examiner stops you—asks you to summarize your findings.

You summarise: You have examined John, a one-year-old boy. He appears small. He is jaundiced. There is a large abdominal scar in the upper abdomen extending across. He also has non-tender hepatomegaly and splenomegaly–both approximately 3 cm below costal margin. He has left inguinal hernia and swelling of right testicle – you can get over. He has no clubbing or cyanosis and is quite active interacting with you

You do not need to stop and can move on to your impression:

In your opinion John has had surgery—most likely for biliary atresia but would like to ask mother some questions.

Examiner allows you one questions: Was John operated for being jaundiced (yellow) after 3 months of age? She agrees and adds it was at 4 months.

The ensuing discussion with the examiner is highlighted in the next section.

What is expected from the candidate?
- Introduces self to the mother and requests verbal consent.
- Makes it known that hand hygiene has been done before touching the patient.
- Enquires whether John is well.
- Keeps the patient at ease and keeps explaining to Ms Baby what the candidate is doing.
- Has examined for icterus in natural sunlight by taking child to the window.
- Examines patient lying flat on the couch.
- Kneels down by the side of the couch and do not stoop over the patient.
- Detects the abdominal scars and able to explain that the bigger scar is due to the Kasai procedure and the smaller scars can be explained by a biopsy and abdominal drain post-surgery.
- Keeps eye on the face to detect any tenderness.
- Provides a realistic measure of the hepatomegaly and splenomegaly by finger breadths but should be ready to measure it formally if advised by the examiner.

- Demonstrates percussion to find liver dullness and establish hepatomegaly and completes.
- The candidate should be able to correlate the findings of an Asian child with jaundice, hepatomegaly and splenomegaly to Biliary atresia followed by a Kasai procedure.

The discussion with the candidate may include:

- Biliary atresia is more common in children of Asian and Afro-Caribbean origin.
- Presents with pale or clay coloured stool and prolonged conjugated hyperbilirubinaemia.
- Kasai procedure is more successful if done within first 6 weeks of life.
- Liver transplantation is often necessary by 2 years of age
- Differential diagnosis to consider in John's case would be Galactosemia, Glycogen storage disorder.
- Regular follow-up with a paediatrician, gastroenterologist, hepatologist, dietitian necessary.

ABDOMINAL EXAMINATION—CHRONIC RENAL FAILURE

Information given to the candidate

You are the candidate. On entering the room the examiner introduces you to Henry, a 14-year-old boy. He is sitting on the examination couch.

You are asked to examine the abdominal Henry. You are allowed to talk to the patient but not allowed to take history from him unless specified by the examiner.

Henry looks well.

You have 9 minutes. There will be a warning bell at 7 min. (UP)

Examination

Introduce yourself to Henry. Inform him of what you have been asked to do and ask for his consent for examining him.

Take the opportunity to look around and also carry out a quick general examination including eyes, lymph gland, hands, dysmorphic feature, nutritional status, TPN lines, scratch marks, oedema, etc.

You find
• He is short for his age
• He is pale
• A scar in the right arm
• On touching it you think it is an arteriovenous fistula

You ask him to lie down.

On inspection from the bed end: You note
• A scar on the abdomen, near left flank approaching the back.
• Abdominal distension
• Visible para umbilical veins
• Umbilical hernia.

On palpation after informing Henry that—"I am going to feel your tummy". Keep looking at his face while palpating for signs of pain or discomfort.
• No organomegaly.
• Check for ascites by percussion/shifting dullness.
• Listening to bowel sound, renal bruits.
• No swelling or tenderness on the back
• Genital—Normal, no oedema,
• No hernia—Inguinal or femoral.

Turn to examiner and summarise your finding:

Henry 14-year-old looks well and comfortable. He looks small for his age and I would like to plot his height and weight on appropriate growth chart. He looks pale. There is no jaundice, oedema, clubbing or lymphadenopathy. He has a scar in his right wrist and a tortuous arterio-venous fistula there. He also has a scar in his left flank extending to his back. His abdomen is soft, non tender, there is no hepatosplenomegaly and the bowel sounds are normal.

These clinical signs suggest Henry has chronic renal failure. He has had surgery and needs or has needed renal dialysis in the past. His abdominal scar can be due to possible nephrectomy.

What is expected from the candidate
- Introduce to Henry, seek verbal consent for examination.
- Follow hand hygiene
- Keep the patient comfortable and build a rapport.
- Identify pallor, short stature, scar at he wrist, abdominal scar
- Correlate the hand finding with AV fistula
- Correlate AV fistula with need for haemodialysis.
- Identify signs of chronic renal failure i.e. short stature, pale complexion, fistula for dialysis, possible nephrectomy scar.
- Basic management of chronic renal failure including:
- Medication, controlling hypertension, renal osteodystrophy, possibility of future renal transplant, etc.

Supporting care for chronic disease may need to be discussed:
- Mental health support by Child psychiatry,
- Educational support,
- Support for parents and other siblings in the family.

Comments: Chronic renal failure
MCUG—Reflux uropathy hydronephrosis

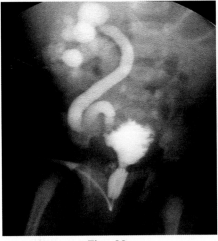

Fig. 30

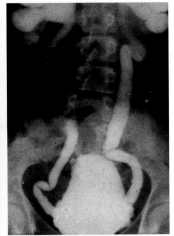

Fig. 31

Reflux is associated with 5–25% of end stage renal failure in childhood worldwide.

Likelihood of renal damage: Age at onset of first infection/prolonged exposure to recurrent infections/biological host factors/bacterial virulence.

More likely if there are structural/functional abnormalities

Reference

Children with Chronic Renal Failure In Sweden. Paediatric Nephrology, 1990, 4, 249–52 http://guidance.nice.org.uk/CG54/SlideSet/ppt/English NICE guidelines CG54 for UTI and renal failure.

Investigations following Childhood UTI, Medicine in Practice, vol 2, no 2, April 1995

ABDOMINAL EXAMINATION: NEPHRECTOMY

Information given to the candidate

You are a candidate and on entering the room you are introduced to Henry, a 14-year-old boy by the examiner.

Examiner asks you to examine his abdomen.

You are allowed to talk to the patient but not allowed to take history from him unless specified by the examiner.

You have 9 minutes. There will be a warning bell at 7 min (UP).

Examination

Introduce yourself to Henry and take the opportunity to look around.

General examination: He is short for his age and is pale. In his right arm there is a scar and when you feel a thrill—suggestive of an AV fistula.

You further note
- A scar in the abdomen near left flank approaching the back.
- No abdominal distension,
- No visible organomegaly,
- No caput medusae,
- No hernia.

You proceed towards palpation and it is a good practice to inform him that—I am going to feel your tummy. Keep looking at his face while palpating.
- No organomegaly.
- Percussion for ascites—none
- Bowel sound—normal.
- No renal bruits.

Do not forget to examine the back for swelling, tenderness, etc.
Ask permission to look for genitals, anal orifice, hernial orifices.
Ask to plot his height and weight in the growth chart.

Turn to examiner and summarise your findings:

Henry 14-year-old looks well and comfortable. He looks small for his age but I would like to plot him in growth chart. He is pale but no jaundice, oedema, clubbing, lymphadenopathy is noted. He has a scar in his right hand and a tortuous AV fistula in his right arm. He has a scar in his left flank and back. His abdomen is soft non-tender with no hepatosplenomegaly with normal bowel sounds. He does not have any evidence of chronic liver disease.

I think, Henry has signs of chronic renal failure for which he is undergoing hemodialysis and his abdominal scar can be due to possible nephrectomy.

What is expected from the candidate?
- Introduce yourself to Henry and seek verbal consent.
- Follow hand hygiene
- Keep the patient comfortable and try to build a rapport.
- Identify the pallor, short stature, scar in the hand, abdominal scar.
- Correlate the hand finding with AV fistula
- To relate AV fistula with hemodialysis.
- To identify signs of chronic renal failure, i.e. short stature, pale complexion, fistula for dialysis, possible nephrectomy scar.
- Basic management of chronic renal failure includes the medication for controlling hypertension, renal osteodystrophy, possibility of future renal transplant, etc.
- Supporting care in form of DLA, child psychiatry, educational support, support for parents may need to be discussed as well.

Development

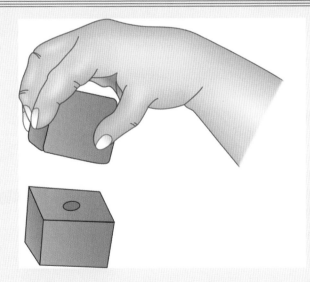

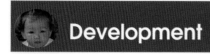
DEVELOPMENTAL ASSESSMENT

THROUGH FIRST YEAR AND TWO

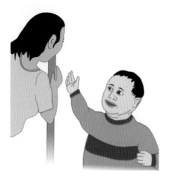

Peak-a-boo—6 months

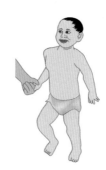

Walking—hand held 10–14 months

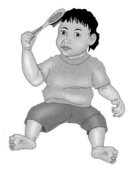

Sitting and imitating 18 months

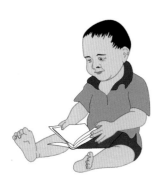

12 months

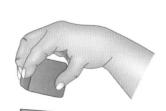

Two cubes—18 months

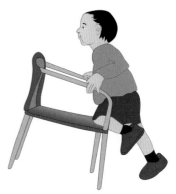

Pulling on to chair—18–24 months

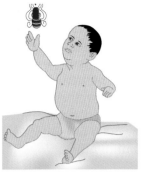

Sitting unsupported reaching out (8–9 months)

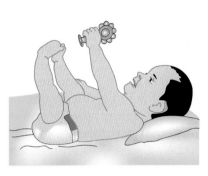

Hand and feet regard 3–4 months

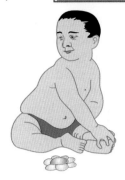

Independent sitting 6–7 months

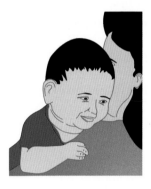

Good head control 3–4 months

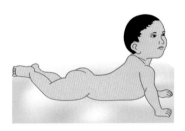

Chest off couch 5–6 months

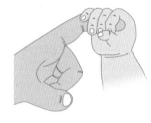

Palmar grasp (6 –7 months)

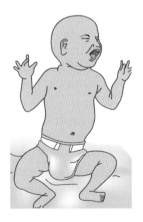

Upset child
Sitting and in nappies

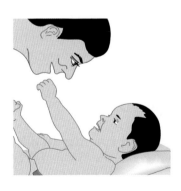

Fixing and smiling 6 weeks

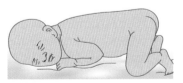

2–4 weeks

The RCPCH gives special importance to development assessment and it is a mandatory station for the membership examination. Candidates often perceive this station as the most difficult. A proper development assessment, even by experienced community paediatricians takes hours hence the college never expects the candidates to do so in seven to nine minutes in exam scenarios. The expectation from the candidates is to be able to demonstrate a well structured examination technique to elicit the age appropriate milestones, i.e. the normative assessment (keeping in mind that performance of a child can be influenced by anxiety, tiredness, etc.) and being able to interpret them confidently.

Thus candidates are expected
1. To be able to identify those children who may not follow the normative stage.
2. To be proficient in rapid assessment of gross motor and fine motor skills.
3. To be able to anticipate and to respond appropriately to age-related behaviour, i.e. separation anxiety.
4. To estimate developmental age that is supported by evidence of the age appropriate skill a child can perform .
5. To observe that a child **is not able to perform a skill which might be expected of a slightly older child.**
6. To be able to discuss appropriate management steps for a child with developmental problems.

   Our aim is to give you some practical and useful tips for this station.
   - Work on and improve your observation skills. This is a station where you have to show the examiner how efficient you are to pick up clues just by watching a child.
   - Try to describe, in your mind, any child that you see. When I was preparing for my exam, I used to practice describing any child I came across. This simple but very useful tip will improve your fluency in describing a child.
   - Develop an approach of mentally observing the child even when you are greeting the examiner and the parent. The first interaction with the child can give you a lot of information, i.e. stranger anxiety, no eye contact, fixity with any object.
   - We would recommend you to describe the patient to your examiner as you go along (until asked to stop/clarify, etc.) which will keep both you and your examiner engaged.
   - Work on targeted questions that you may be allowed to ask parents. Your questions should be clear and specific. Instead of open questions you should be prepared with closed question to save time, i.e. Can he climb stairs? Can she ride a tricycle? Can he drink from a cup?
   - You will have to demonstrate your rapport with children by being able to engage them with blocks, book, bead, crayon, etc. To carry out specific activities.
   - Your instructions should be specific and simple to follow.
   - Ask mother to give the instructions if the child is apprehensive or shy.

- Choose simple objects like **books, beads, blocks, ball, paper and crayon.**
- Practice with these tools with any child you come across (work or home). Use simple commands like "Would you like to play?" "Let us make a tower with these coloured blocks", "Can you make a tower like me", etc.
- Do not be fixed with one object. If he does not like blocks move on to something else.
- **Do not lose the child's attention and do not let him get bored.**
- Always take **only one tool at a time so as not to divert attention and** remove it from sight when you wish to move on to next tool.

Remember patterns of development progress are from simple to complex, from head to toe, from inner to outer and from simple actions to more complex actions, e.g. children sit before standing and then run or skip. Physical control and coordination begins with a child's head and develops down the body through the arms, hands and back and finally to legs and feet. Development proceeds from actions nearer the body to more complex ones further from the body. For example, children can co-ordinate their arms, using gross motor skills to reach for an object, before they have learned the fine motor skills necessary to use their fingers to pick it up. Development progresses from general responses to specific ones. For example, a young baby shows pleasure by a massive general response—the eyes widen, and the legs and arms move vigorously whereas an older child shows pleasure by smiling or using appropriate words or gestures.

Development is described grossly as:
- Physical
- Sensory
- Cognitive and language
- Emotional and social

Physical development —2 main domains
- Gross motor skill—sitting, walking, running, climbing, etc.
- Fine motor skill
  - Gross manipulative skills (throwing, catching, etc.)
  - Fine manipulative skills (pincer, drawing, using spoon, doing buttons, etc).

Sensory development is the process by which we receive information through the senses, i.e. vision, hearing, smell, touch, taste and proprioception.

Cognitive and language development
- Cognitive—recognising, reasoning, knowing, and understanding.
- Perception—when we make sense of what we see, hear, touch, smell and taste.
- This is affected by previous experiences and knowledge.

Language development—development of communication skill, i.e.
- Receptive speech—what a person understands
- Expressive speech—the words the person produces
- Articulation—the person's actual pronunciation of words.
- Please remember that receptive speech develops earlier than expressive speech

Emotional and social development
- Emotional development—awareness of oneself, feeling towards other people, developing self-esteem and self concept.
- Social development—child's relationship with other people. Socialisation is the process of learning skills and attitude that help the child to live easily with other members of the community.

In exam the development station usually comes with one of the three tasks.

The first task

In my exam I was introduced to Tom, a fourteen month old boy who was going for kidney transplant. **My task was to assess his developmental age and comment if it was appropriate for his chronological age.** Here in seven minutes the task would be to assess all the parameters and not going into too many details. For example, as I saw him walking around the room trying to go to a nearby shelf, I knew he was already 13 months plus. Taking the examiners permission I asked mother that if he can run, climb stairs, etc. and I got to know about his gross motor skills. Similarly giving him crayons and paper and observing what he did with it gave me a rough idea regarding his fine motor skills. If he was not interested in crayons I could give him a book which would show his ability to turn the pages and his verbal ability. By responding to his name he gave me a clue about his language development. I asked mother about finger food, drinking from cup, level of toilet training, etc. Finally a quick comment about vision and hearing which I already knew from my interaction with the child. So although it might look daunting to do this station in 7 minutes, in reality I could assess and comment his developmental age was appropriate for his chronological age.

In a clinic a paediatrician should be able to grossly identify if a child's development is age appropriate or not.

A quick tip: If you concentrate on what a child **cannot do** in fixing a developmental age it might work better. We have given some example but you can formulate your own parameters with tools you choose to use in the exam.

For example
- In gross motor assessment—Thomas:
  Cannot skip or hop: <5 yr
  Cannot ride a tricycle: <3 yr
  Cannot run freely: <2 yr
  Cannot walk steadily: <1 yr
  Cannot sit without support: <6 mth
  Cannot support head control :< 3 mth?
- In fine motor with the crayons—Thomas:
  Cannot copy a Δ: < 5 yr
  Cannot copy a □ : < 4 yr

Cannot copy a ○ : < 3 yr
Cannot copy a + : < 2 y
Cannot imitate–strokes: < 1 yr

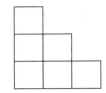

- With the blocks—Thomas:
  Cannot copy 3 stair patterns with 6 blocks: < 4–5 yr
  Cannot copy a bridge or tower with 10 blocks: < 3 yr
  Cannot copy a tower of six blocks: < 2 yr
  Cannot copy a tower of 3–4 blocks: < 18 mth
  Cannot copy tower of 2 blocks: < 12 mth
- Speech and language—Thomas:
  Cannot say his birthday or name 4 colours : < 5 yr
  Cannot say full address, count up to 20: < 4 yr
  Cannot say age, sex, count up to 10: <3 yr
  Cannot form 3 word sentences,
  Cannot follow simple instructions, i.e. Will you get me the ball: **<2 yr**
  Cannot point to named body parts, simple word like baba dada, etc.: **<12 mth**

The second task
You may be asked to assess any single parameter of development. Usually speech and language or fine motor skills is asked to be assessed. This task will need a different approach. Often you may be told a child's age, alternatively, you may be asked to comment on his developmental age. You should have a **well rehearsed and structured approach** to complete this task.

Some useful tips
- Always have a few tools ready—**books, blocks, beads**. The child may not be interested in blocks but may engage with books.
- We suggest:
  - Do not repeatedly try to make him do things which he is not keen to. You may well lose his attention and interest.
  - Do not keep a number of tools/objects scattered as that will distract the child.
  - Once you get the child engaged with blocks or books keep challenging him as far as possible.
  - Do not try to make the child do **all the tasks you have learnt**. Your aim here is to arrive at his development age rather than make the child do the entire task which is practically never achievable.

The Third task
Your task may be asked to comment on a child's **developmental status**. In this task usually the child has global development delay or is an autistic child. Again

a holistic approach is needed. Normative assessments should be supported with observations; observing is an essential skill for anyone working with children. If you are dealing with an autistic child the examiner will be fully aware that in a 5–7 min station it is almost impossible to arrive at a diagnosis but they would like you to pick up some clues like unusual ways of playing, repetitive body movement, hyperactive behaviour, etc.

Later in this chapter we will have a few case based discussions.

Details of the normative assessment are available to you in many textbooks. In the appendix we give you a quick reference range for each area that you can use as a skeleton to build on in your preparation.

The guru mantra for fluency is regular practise.

You need to demonstrate an organised approach to developmental assessment and the best thing you can do to improve your skills is to assess as many children as possible.

- Start with children who are cooperative and do not have any evident developmental delay. Follow a clear and systematic pattern.
- Try to do all of this with the child sitting at a small table.
- Clear all items from the work surface away.
- Bring out one tool/item at a time.
- Remove the item from sight each time before moving on to the next one.
- Do not leave lots of different items on the table to distract the child—**a recipe for disaster**.

Show the examiners that you have done this before and understand what you would expect of the child. If the child is unable to perform / complete the task set—make things simpler and comment on the gaps in ability.

Within each developmental category it should be possible for you to define developmental age within 2–3 months before 2 years of age and within 4–6 months between 2 and 5 years of age. Interpretation of the developmental assessment should be made with regard to the range of normal findings and in the context of a child's illness or other associated condition.

Trainees who have experience of community paediatrics are at an advantage in terms of developmental assessments, knowledge of support in community and various allowances available but in reality that is not mandatory. You can improve your skills with regular practise with children you come across and attending community paediatric sessions. Practice developmental assessment every day with at least one child. More you interact with children and are able to engage them with blocks, crayons or books to complete set tasks, your confidence and familiarity will be reflected in the exam.

While preparing for the exam arrange to attend, as many sessions as feasible, at your local child development centre (CDC) for an overview. Spend time with multidisciplinary teams, consultants in their clinics, physiotherapists and occupational therapists during various sessions. Observe, make mental and physical notes and have any doubts clarified. If possible carry out developmental assessment in their presence and get a feedback. Remember—your performance can only get better.

You may be tasked by the examiner to assess vision and/or hearing for different age groups. Although these are less likely but be well prepared and update your theoretical knowledge.

Children with special needs may have concerns/difficulties with:
- Physical impairment—problem with mobility, coordination, articulation (dyspraxia)
- Sensory impairment—sight/hearing
- Speech/language difficulties—delay/articulation/stuttering.
- Learning disabilities-moderate to severe.
- Specific learning disability—dyslexia (reading), writing/numeracy.
- Emotional difficulties—autism, anxiety, fear, depression.
- Behavioural difficulties—attention deficit hyperactivity disorder, aggression.
- Medical condition—asthma, cystic fibrosis, diabetes, chronic renal failure, etc
- Global developmental disorder—Down syndrome, Rett's syndrome, cerebral palsy, etc.

Providing care for children with special needs:

Child development centre (CDC)—Doctor, therapists, health visitor, social worker work together in **Multi-disciplinary team** to provide necessary care.

Specialist help
a. Physiotherapy
b. Speech and language therapy
c. Occupational therapy
d. Home learning scheme, i.e. portage
e. Equipment and special aid
f. Financial support—personal care/mobility, etc.
g. Toy libraries
h. Specialist play groups, opportunity groups, children's centres respite care
i. Nurseries, school nurseries, classes.

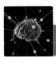

Remember !

Keep the child engaged and one tool or toy at a time
Avoid distraction by removing from field of vision
Focussed questions in uncooperative child—with permission

SPEECH DELAY—ISOLATED

Information given to the candidate

You are the candidate and on entering the station, the examiner introduces you to Ava, a 3-year-old. She has been referred by her GP to the paediatric team as there were concerns regarding her speech from the staff at her nursery.

Your task is: Can you assess her speech development.

You have 9 minutes. There will be a warning bell at 7 min. (UP)

Examination

You introduce yourself to Ava's mother and obtain her consent, inform of hand hygiene. You greet Ava.

You note

- Ava is sitting at one corner of the room. She is holding a pencil using her thumb and first two fingers and trying to draw something. She looks apprehensive and moves closer to her mother as you approach Ava. You introduce yourself to mother and to Ava. She looks shy. You approach the table and ask her name. She does not reply you. On your behalf her mother asks her name. She mumbles which you cannot understand.

At this stage you can ask mother to choose a book for Ava which she might be interested in.

- You show the book to Ava. She seems to be interested. You point to different objects in the book and ask her if she knows them. She still does not answer you. You once again take mothers help. She responds to her mother and starts naming the objects.
- You note she has got a good vocabulary. Gradually she responds to you and answers simple question like show me the cat, what the baby is doing, etc.
- You note she knows the basic colors and she can count 10 objects from the picture book. Slowly Ava becomes chatty and carries on a conversation with you.
- You note Ava has a good vocabulary but there is a problem with articulation as she pronounces dog as "og", door as "or". Water as "oter".
- You ask mother if she is aware of this. Mother says her health visitor has referred her to speech specialist for this.
- Looking at the paper you see that she was drawing a man with eyes and lips.

You check with mother about

- Ava's gross motor skill, i.e. if she can ride tricycle, climb stairs.
- Mother informs you that she is toilet trained
- She eats with spoon and fork
- Drinks from her own cup.

After checking with examiner you briefly ask mother about her birth history, any h/o tongue tie, significant past medical history or any family history specially related to speech problems.

During this conversation you note Ava goes to the corner of the room where she discovers a doll and excitedly calls her mother and points to the doll. Mother calls her by name and she runs toward her with that doll and hugs her.

You turn toward the examiner and summarizes your findings:
Ava is a lovely 3-year-old girl. She does not have any dysmorphic features. She does not have a hearing aid. She is interested in toys and pictures. She responds to her name. She can name basic colours. She has a good vocabulary. Her receptive speech is age appropriate as she understands simple instructions and responds appropriately. She has difficulty with her articulation as she is struggling with pronunciation of certain words.

Although I did not formally assess her other developmental parameters but they seem to be age appropriate as she can ride a tricycle, she can draw a circle and she can also feed herself. She interacts with her mother very well. She does not have any obvious problem with vision and hearing.

To conclude Ava has isolated speech articulation difficulty and I would refer her to speech and language team for formal assessment.

What is expected from the candidate?

- Introduces self to the mother and Ava and requests verbal consent.
- Makes it known that hand hygiene has been done before touching the patient.
- Personal observation even before rapport formation.
- Keeps the patient at ease and gives simple and easy to understand commands.
- To build rapport with the patient.
- To take the mothers help while assessment.
- To choose correct tool for examination, i.e. book.
- Ability to check hearing and understanding of the patient.
- Ability to comments on different aspects of speech and language development including receptive, expressive, etc.
- Ability to identify patient's articulation abnormality.
- Ability to assess other parameters briefly before drawing conclusion.
- Addressing parental concern.
- Able to discuss with the examiner about other speech problems and their management and refer her to the SALT (**S**peech **A**nd **L**anguage **T**herapy) team.

CLINICAL PRACTICE NOTES

- Always follow the norm **observation**, assessment, parental concern.
- Building rapport
- Opportunistic examination technique.
- Choose right tool.
- Do not try to too hard to initiate conversation.
- Your patient might completely be withdrawn.
- Involve mother wherever possible.
- Be able to differentiate between different aspects of speech, i.e receptive, expressive, articulation.

Normal Milestones

Parallel play: It is when toddlers play by themselves, standing or sitting next to each other and is typical of most kids around age two.

Group play and sharing does not usually evolve until age three. Until then, most infants and younger toddlers simply play by themselves next to each other, in parallel play.

Ability to ride a tricycle and/or a bicycle is an important milestone that most children can reach by the time they are three years old.

Preschoolers can usually learn to pedal a tricycle once they are about three years old.

By four, they can usually learn to ride a two wheel cycle with training wheels, which they can take off when they are about five to six years old.

Most children can write letters and spell their own name by the time they are five years old.

Most children can count to ten or more once they are four to five and a half years old.

DEVELOPMENT: 14-MONTH-OLD CHILD

Information given to the candidate

On entering the station, the examiner introduces you. Mrs Smith and her son. Joy is 14-month-old boy. He has bilateral obstructive uropathy. He is waiting for his renal transplant soon.

You are asked to assess his developmental milestones.

You have 9 minutes. There will be a warning bell at 7 min. (UP)

Examination

Introduce yourself to Mrs Smith and Joy. You explain and clarify your role. Ask for their consent and inform of hand hygiene. During introductions You note

- Joy is wandering around the room and exploring things.
- Look carefully and comment on his overall appearance (including absence of dysmorphism, big/small head, etc.)

As you note he is steadily walking around you can comment that his gross motor seems appropriate for his age.

With permission from the examiner
Ask his mother if he likes looking at books. If so select an age appropriate book and offer him the book.

- Joy looks interested in that book and tries to pat on the book but does not try to open it.
- You open the book and he points on an object like a ball.
- You can ask him to point to other simple pictures in that page.
- He tries to turn the page.

Next you take the book away and offer him a few blocks. Ask him to copy you. Can you do this? He seems not very keen. Ask mother to do so.

- He can copy 2–3 block towers.

You ask mother to wave bye bye.

- He waves back to mother. When you call him by name he responds to it.

Ask examiner if you are allowed to ask mother some information regarding personal social life, i.e. Can Joy drink from a beaker? Can he tell that he is wet? Does he like finger food?

Turn towards examiner and summarise your finding: Joy is a 14-month-old, looks alert, active and playful. There are no obvious dysmorphic features. He can walk steadily. He can do a 3 block tower. He cannot turn pages yet. He responds to his name. He knows and points to a few common objects. He interacts with his mother well. He can drink from his bottle and loves finger food. His vision and hearing seems intact though I would like to get a formal vision and hearing test.

I think his developmental age is appropriate for his chronological age.

What is expected from the candidate?

- Introduce yourself to Joy and his mother.
- Demonstrate hand hygiene.
- Able to gather as many as clues possible from personal observation.
- Follow the norm: Personal observation, personal assessment, parental concern.
- Able to draw inference from observation.

CLINICAL PRACTICE

- Ability to follow clear and systematic pattern
- Ability to demonstrate the tasks to the child
- Show the examiner that you understand what you would expect of the child
- Basic understanding of the normative assessment.

NOTES

Normal development milestones

Rolling over is often one of the first major motor milestones that babies reach by 3–6 months old. Spending less time prone or on their stomach, since the release of the Back to Sleep recommendations to reduce the risk of SIDS, has caused some infants to roll over a little later than they used to though.

It can also cause some delays in picking up other milestones, including sitting up and crawling. Fortunately, by the time they are toddlers, these delays all seem to disappear no matter how a baby sleeps, so it likely more appropriate to describe these kids as having a 'lag' in their development and not a true delay.

Still, most infants roll over when they are between three to six months old, first from their front to their back, and then from their back to their front.

Infants use a thumb-finger pincer grasp, at about 7 to 11 months old, earlier they pick things up with a more immature palmer grasp.

A baby **stand with support** but keep in mind that even once infants can stand with support, they cannot usually pull themselves to a standing position on their own until they are 8 to 10 months old.

An infant takes his/her **first steps** between 11 and 15 months.

Whatever, makes children take the leap from cruising around, to in which they walk while holding on to things, to taking those first steps on their own it happens between 10 and 16 months?

Is it courage, balance, or just chance?

Pretend play or imitating activities is a milestone infants reach by 10–16 months old.

Pretend play often involves things like using a computer mouse like a phone, imitating an activity a toddler has seen his parents do over and over.

Toddlers will also begin to copy more of their parents daily household tasks, such as dusting and sweeping, at around 18 months.

Pretend play will get more elaborate as your child gets older; for example, a child pretends he is a doctor, fireman, or race car driver.

DEVELOPMENT : 3½ YEARS OLD—AUTISTIC SPECTRUM

What is expected from the candidate

On entering the station, the examiner introduces you to Bobby and Mrs Jones. Booby is a 3½-year-old has been referred by the audiologist to the paediatric team. He was sent for hearing assessment as there were concerns regarding his hearing. The audiologist has raised certain concerns while trying to perform the hearing test.

Your task is "Can you please examine Bobby and comment on his development."

You have 9 minutes. There will be a warning bell at 7 min. (UP)

Examination

Introduce yourself to Mrs Jones and Bobby. You explain and clarify your role. Ask for their consent and inform of hand hygiene. During introductions

You note
• Bobby is sitting on the floor with his mother.
• He is playing with a car.

You sit beside them. He does not look at you. You ask his name but he does not respond to you. You attempt to engage him in a conversation regarding his car but you do not get any response. He seems too busy to carry on any conversation.

You ask his mother to engage with him. You note that he responds to his mother but still does not look at you. His mother turns him towards you. He does not have any hearing aid. He does not have any obvious dysmorphic features. He continues to look at his car and plays with the wheels. He ignores you completely.

At this stage you try to show him a book. He does not seem interested.

You ask the mother to show him the book. Mother says that it is very difficult to divert his attention. She also tells you that he gets really upset if you try to take his car away.

With examiner's permission you ask mother some relevant questions.
• Ask about her concern regarding Bobby.
• Are there any concern with his hearing.
• Check his other developmental parameters like running, riding bike, scribbling.
• Her view of his vocabulary.
• Ask if he can point.
• Enquire about his play, interaction with parents, siblings.

- Any other concerns.
- Relevant medical history (e.g. seizures), any significant birth history.
- Chronological development history to identify any delay in any of the parameters.

There is a knock to alert 7 minutes.

You turn and summarise your finding to the examiner:

Bobby is a 3½-year-old boy sitting comfortably with his mother. He does not have any obvious dysmorphic features. His hearing seems fine as he does not have any hearing aid and he did respond to his mother. He seems engrossed with his car. He is not interested in his surroundings. He did not have any eye contact with me or the examiner. He did not take any interest in any other toys or books. From the history obtained from mother, his gross motor and fine motor parameters seems fine. His mother also informed that he does not like new friends, plays alone for hours and get upset if his routine is altered. His speech is significantly delayed. He does not point yet and usually drags his mother to the object he wants.

To conclude Bobby seems to have gross expressive speech delay most probably associated with a behavioural problem like autistic spectrum disorder for which I would like to refer him to child development centre for formal assessment.

What is expected from the candidate?
- Introduces self to the mother and Bobby and requests verbal consent.
- Makes it known that hand hygiene has been done before touching the patient.
- Personal observation, assessment, parental concerns
- Try to build rapport with the patient.
- To take the mothers help with assessment.
- To choose the correct tool for examination, i.e. book.
- Ability to check hearing and understanding of the patient.
- Ability to comment on Bobby's problem by simply observing him.
- Ability to identify patient's difficulty with expressive speech
- Addressing parental concern.
- Able to discuss with the examiner about autism and its spectrum.

CLINICAL PRACTICE NOTES

Primarily you should use information from direct observation of the child and take clues from:
1. Unusual way of playing
2. Lack of imaginative play.
3. Repetitive body movements
4. Hyperactive behaviour

5. Unusual use of pronouns, echolalia
   - Candidates may use history from the examiner and the parents to explore the child's behavioural development.
   - Gross idea about social interaction and play patterns in different age groups.
   - Basic knowledge about autism and autistic spectrum disorder including Asperger's syndrome (a rare developmental disorder which impairs a child's understanding of, and her/his ability to relate to, the environment.)
   - Outline the management plan, i.e. CDC referral, parent and child behavioural therapy, disability allowance, support to the parents, etc. **(keep in mind this is a lifelong disability of social interaction.)**

DEVELOPMENT: PREMATURE CHILD

Information given to the candidate

You are the candidate and on entering the examiner introduces you to Skye, now aged 8½ month. She was born at 27 weeks of gestation. Currently she is reported to be well.

Her mother, Ms Goodwin, has come for a check up as she is worried that Skye sometimes does not fix and follow when tired.

You are requested to do a full developmental examination

You are allowed to talk to Ms Goodwin but is not allowed to ask any history.

You have 9 minutes to complete the station; a warning bell will be given at 7 minutes. (SP)

The examination

You introduce yourself to Ms Goodwin and explain that you are going to examine how Skye responds to various stimuli and thus assess her development. You let the examiner and Ms Goodwin know that hand hygiene has been observed.

While Ms Goodwin undresses Skye you note:
• She looks well, smiles responsibly and making cooing noises.
• Small whitish dots over the dorsum of hands and feet.
• Appears small for her age and offer to formally plot her on a growth chart.

You test the **vision:**
• You request Ms Goodwin and the examiner that you will need silence to demonstrate the vision.
• You take a bright red ball and show it to Skye and then move it in the midline and then up and down. Skye follows the ball in all directions.
• You do not see any nystagmus.

You explain to the examiner know that Skye is fixing and following well both in midline and also up and down.

You then test **Hearing:**
• You take a rattle and make gentle noise and Skye turns towards the noise both sides.
• Skye also responded when Ms Goodwin called her name.

You then tell the examiner that Skye appears to hear well however being premature you will prefer a formal hearing assessment to be done on her. You then go to assess **fine motor development:**
• You offer the rattle to Skye and she grabs it nicely.
• You offer another toy to her and she reaches to take it in the other hand. Did not demonstrate hand dominance.

- The examiner is made aware of the findings.

You then explain to Ms Goodwin that you are going to see what Skye does when lifted, made to sit, etc.; thus demonstrate **gross motor development**:
- You gently pull Skye up by her hands
- She sat momentarily without support with a hunched back, for a longer time with support.
- You lift her by holding her under her arm pits and feel that Skye has got good truncal tone.
- While put on her front she lifts her head and holds it there and looks around.

You ask the examiner whether you can ask Ms Goodwin a few **questions** and you are allowed two.
- You ask Ms Goodwin whether Skye is rolling over—trying but not there as yet.
- Does Skye recognise her—Ms Goodwin replied in the affirmative.

You then offer to put the dress back for Skye but Ms Goodwin took over, you thank her.

You now summarise your findings: You explain that Skye has sequel of a premature baby but fixing and following properly, listens ok, uses both hand, sitting with support and reported to be trying to roll over which will put her at a developmental age of 5 to 6 months.

You are then asked what you would say to Ms Goodwin about her concerns and you explain that Skye demonstrated that she can fix and follow properly and young babies like Skye sometimes not do so properly when they are tired.

The ensuing discussion is highlighted in the next section.

What is expected from the candidate?
- Introduces self to the carer (Ms Goodwin) and requests verbal consent.
- Makes it known that hand hygiene has been done before touching the patient.
- Keeps the patient at ease.
- Observes silence while testing vision.
- Explains limitation of the hearing assessment and informs that a formal hearing test is necessary in this scenario. Demonstrates use of both hands. Gently pulls the child to sit and then lifts up the child, does not cause distress to the child.
- Offers to dress Skye up at the end of the session.
- Asks relevant questions when allowed.
- Candidate is able to patch up all the findings and say that the development appears appropriate for Skye's corrected age.
- Candidate may offer to do a full neurological examination in view of the history of prematurity.

GENERAL NOTE

It is important to know the developmental milestones for different age group. It is very important that you remain opportunistic and observant while trying to do the development in young children. The scheme should be:

1. Try and engage the child yourself
2. Involve the parents
3. Ask questions after seeking permission from the examiner (as a last resort).

DEVELOPMENT: MOTOR DEVELOPMENT OF AN INFANT WITH DOWN'S SYNDROME

Information given to the candidate

You are the candidate and on entering the station, the examiner introduces you to Thomas, a 9-month-old boy with Down's syndrome. He is sitting on the floor with his mother Ms Blackburn and playing.

You are requested to examine for his motor developmental.

You are allowed to talk to Ms Blackburn but is not allowed to ask any history unless allowed by the examiner.

You have 9 minutes to complete the station; a warning bell will be given at 7 minutes (SP).

The examination

You introduce yourself to Ms Blackburn and explain that you are going to play with Thomas to find how he is developing for his movements and activities. You let the examiner and Ms Blackburn know that hand hygiene has been observed.

You observe Thomas
- Can see and hear very well.
- His growth appears normal for his age
- He has features suggestive of Down's syndrome.

Thomas is playing alone on the floor and you **sit down beside him** and start assessing his **motor development**:
- He easily engages with you.
- He is sitting with a straight back
- You offer him two cubes and he takes two cubes and happily and bangs them together.
- You offer a 3rd cube and at this point you notice that he tries transfer the cube to his other hand although he does not manage two cubes in one hand.
- He is using both hands equally with no hand dominance.
- You then offer a rattle at a distance and he reaches for it keeping his balance well maintained.
- You request Ms Blackburn to call him and he manages to crawl towards her and pulls himself to stand holding onto mother's knees.

The **fine motor development** is further tested now
- You tear a paper into few small pieces, roll and offer these to Thomas. You notice that Thomas manages to pick these up with a coarse pincer grasp.
- You then offer a plastic cup to him and he mages to pick it up well and tries to bring it to his mouth but ends up banging it on his forehead.
- Similar observation was noted with a spoon as well.

At this point the examiner allows you to ask couple of questions to mum and then summarise your findings.

You **ask** Ms Blackburn
- Can Thomas roll over both ways—the answer is he does so.
- You then ask about finger foods and you receive a positive response about this as well.

You summarize: Thomas engaged with you quite well and playing with him.

Gross motor findings were that Thomas demonstrated crawling, pulling to stand, sitting unaided, keeping balance and rolling over as reported by his mother when reaching for things which will be consistent with his biological age of 9 months.

The fine motor findings noted were a coarse pincer grasp, banging cubes together, trying to put a cup and spoon to his mouth and finger feeds as reported by his mother which will again be consistent with his biological age of 9 months.

At this point mum volunteered that she has got no concerns about Thomas' development thus far and this fact was also reiterated by the paediatrician at the Child Development Centre last week.

The ensuing discussion is highlighted in the next section.

What is expected from the candidate?
- Introduces self to the mother Ms Blackburn and requests verbal consent.
- Makes it known that hand hygiene has been done before touching the patient.
- Keeps Thomas at ease and sits down beside him and try to engage him in playing.
- Demonstrates use of both hands and keeps the play area tidy so that Thomas does not get distracted
- Involves Ms Blackburn at the later part of the assessment to demonstrate that Thomas can do more in a familiar environment in presence of his mother.
- Demonstrates pincer grasp.
- Asks relevant questions when allowed.
- Candidate is able to patch up all the findings and say that the motor development appears appropriate for Thomas' age.
- Candidate may offer to do a full neurological examination in view of the history of Down's syndrome and should be aware about the need for long term developmental follow-up in such a child.
- Offer to formally plot Thomas on a Down's children growth chart.

GENERAL NOTE

It is very important that you remain opportunistic and observant while trying to do the development in young children or infants. In the scenario that you have just read the motor development was assessed as a whole to start with. It is important to keep noticing what the child can or cannot do as the child may have demonstrated something which you planned to examine at a later stage but the child had become reluctant by then. These have been discussed in details at the start of this section.

Focused History and Management Planning

A wise old owl sat in an oak'
The more he heard, the less he spoke;
The less he spoke, the more he heard;
Why aren't you like that wise old bird? (Anon)

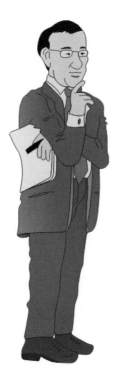 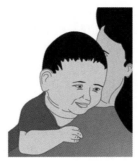

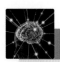

Remember!

Focus on the task given
Include relevant social / family / educational issues
Prioritise management plan as you work through history

The aim of this station is to assess the candidate's ability to take a focussed history, identify key issues, prioritise, able to summarise and formulate a management plan. The task given is specific and candidates will be marked down for getting irrelevant information.

This station has 'replaced' the traditional "long case" except there is no physical examination during this exercise. However, the station is not intended to be a diagnostic exercise. Appropriate interaction with the child and parents is expected. The cases generally have ongoing management problems (chronic disease) or how to approach a new patient in the clinic environment with specific or nonspecific symptoms.

The station is of 22 minutes, 13 minutes with the patient and parents and then 9 minutes with the examiner discussing, scoring points.

You, the candidate, will be given the setting, relevant background information and a specific task. The patient may have a number of comorbidites that may or may not be relevant.

'Focused' does _not_ mean skipping differential diagnosis.

History taking can be either **patient centred** or doctor centred. Doctor centred history taking consists of getting answers to closed questions that relate to symptoms of different systems in usually a predetermined order and thus may not keep the patients perspective on the details of disease.

History taking or data gathering is also as much an exercise of your communication skills. It is important you develop a rapport with the patient. Remember this can easily be damaged by asking inappropriate questions.

Taking a focussed history from a teenager with cystic fibrosis who is being seen for recent weight loss, it will be inappropriate to ask about his birth history. If something specific has to be asked, put it in context.

The history taking should always be developmentally appropriate for the patient's age.

Four main groups being

- Infant
- School age
- Toddler
- Teenager

For teenagers besides other information also ask: **HEADS**

H: home life
E: education
A: activities
D: drugs
S: sex (if appropriate and you feel comfortable in asking)

The following points should also be kept in mind:

Familiarisation: You will need some basic information about the patient at your history and management station. This will be provided and you should digest the information in 2–3 minutes before seeing the 'patient'. You need to mentally go through the next few minutes of the 'consultation', think of the differentials diagnosis and the questions you may be asking. It is acceptable to make brief aide memoire during the 4 minutes.

Rapport: Try and control your nerves. Introduce yourself, address and greet the patient or carer appropriately. Clarify your 'task' so as to minimise the potential to start off on the 'wrong foot'.

Take note of the appearance, behaviour, body language and other features of the 'patient' and any other clues available.

I do not wish to be prescriptive and suggest you do follow what comes naturally to you but the following Opening questions seem to work well:

Thank you for coming. I am Dr XX.
- You can 'paraphrase' the information you have been given and ......
- Your reason for coming today was ....?
- What can I do for you today?
- How may I help you?

(pause, inviting response)

Information gathering: The patient is then encouraged to give details in their own words. **Try and not interrupt** but give lots of encouraging noises and phrases:
- Yes, I see......
- Ummm.....
- OK......
- Tell me more—to expand on the presenting complaint or other information

Your body language needs to be open and receptive, show your interest in the patient and their problems.
- Eye contact is essential
- React to verbal and nonverbal cues

Exploring ideas, concerns and expectations (ICE)

A simile I picked up: Following your initial interview, you should be able to gather enough information so as to change the 'passport' portrait of the individual to a 'family photograph'. The patient does does *not* live in isolation and the illness affects the whole family and management decisions thus far and into the future will need to take account of the whole family.

Patient's **I**deas, **C**oncerns and **E**xpectations are central to any disease process and its good management to explore their thoughts, worries and hopes. This will yield clues to the social and psychological aspects of their problem.

Exploring ICE at the right time—on cues and not at a set time with emphasis on **'You—the patient'.**

This approach will help:
- Improve communication with the 'patient'
- In problem solving
- Discuss and reach a management plan
- Provide reassurance—that **there is a solution and help is available**

It is wise to ask a patient their expectations than to assume you know.

Anchor statements: Station 6—focused history

	Expected standard/Clear pass	Pass	Bare fail	Clear fail	Unacceptable
Part A: Rapport	Full greeting and introduction	Adequately performed but not fully fluent in conducting interview	Incomplete or hesitant greeting and introduction	Significant components omitted or not achieved	Dismissive of parent/child concerns.
	Clarifies role and agrees aims and objectives		Inadequate identification of role, aims objectives.		Fails to put and parent or child at ease
	Good eye contact and posture. perceived to be actively listening (nod etc.) with verbal and non-verbal cues		Poor eye contact and posture. Not perceived to be actively listening (nod etc.) with verbal and non-verbal cues.		
	Appropriate level of confidence. Empathetic nature. Putting parent/child at ease		Does not show appropriate level of confidence, empathetic nature or putting parent/child at ease		
Part A: Focused History	Ask clear question pertinent to the case.	Question reasonable and covers essential issues but omits	Misses relevant information, which would make a difference to management if known	Ask irrelevant questions, poorly understood by	Questions totally unrelated to the problem presented
	Open and closed questions. Patent, child and examiner can hear and understand fully	Occasional essential points	Excessive use of closed question		
			Occasional use of jargon	Excessive use of jargon	Shows no regard to the child/parent.
	Appropriate answers to parents questions	Overall approach structured	Summary incomplete	Does not seek the view of parent/child	No summary
	Structured question. Avoid jargons picks up verbal and non-verbal cues	Appropriate style of questioning		Very poor summary	
	Succinct summary of key issues	Main points summarised			
Part B: Summary management planning and closure	Invites further questions. Summaries.	Summaries most of the important points and suggests best management strategy	Incomplete summary of problem and inadequately	Poor summary	Abrupt ending
	Gives accurate information		Does not relate management to child/parents needs of concerns	Patient unsure of future plans	Inaccurate information given
	Explores options for management	Provides some information about other Services and future plan	Inadequate attempt to determine child/parent understanding	Poor discussion of management options	Lack of regard safe, ethical and effective treatments
	Provides appropriate further contact				

Common complaint against doctors is that we *do not* listen to our patients or their parents. Do Not make this mistake in the exam also.

Listen to what is being said and then summarise it back.

Active listening and suggestions:

Listen carefully to what the patient has told you and do not ask for that information again. You may clarify your understanding of the same by paraphrasing it.

Patient: 'We have come to see you as my daughter, Lucy, is not eating and losing weight.' 'She is missing a lot of school as she is tired all the time'. 'I am worried'. 'She is looking forward to her school trip but I am not sure if I should send her.'

Doctor: 'What are your concerns' will be a bad choice of words—suggest you have not be listening.

"Are you worried?" or "What do you think is wrong with you?" will not go down well.

But "I can see you are worried. Do you have and ideas as to what may be wrong that you may have discussed with your family members or noted on internet?" may get them to open up and come out with their concerns that you can further explore.

In summary remember the following mantra:

Previous knowledge
(details given before you get to see the patient)
(Think through differentials and questions you may ask)
↓
Presenting complaint
↓
Patient gives details in their words
(open questions, clarifications, acting on cues, show interest)
↓
Specific questions
(closed questions with Yes/No answers or specific details)
↓
Ideas, Concerns, Expectations (ICE)
↓
Summarise and ask for clarifications if any
(candidate)

The anchor statement for the station gives the basis for how your performance will be mark. It is available on the web or RCPCH website. Study it carefully. Make a note of the expected standard for a clear pass.

Please remember

Full greetings – clarify role – agree aims and objectives – good *eye* contact – confident approach – clear pertinent open and close questions – avoid jargon – answers parents question appropriately – summary of key issue – invites further questions – ends session with patient smoothly – present good summary and details – accurate information – provide further contacts and information of other agencies as required – concludes and ends smoothly.

Note irrelevant questions, poor rapport with parents or child, excessive technical words that may not be understood by lay people, poor or no summary to parents are all you need to avoid in your clinical practice and on the day!

So practice, practice, practice ....

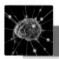

Remember!

Do not 'Lock in' to a specific area at cost of other facets of history
Do not treat it as a communication station
Do not lecture to the patient

HISTORY TAKING AND MANAGEMENT PLANNING: UNPROVOKED SEIZURES

Information given to the candidate: To read before getting into the room
You are in OPD clinic and have the following urgent referral:

Dear Dr

Thank you for seeing Julian, a 7-old-year boy. He was on holidays in Spain with his family last week where he had a generalized convulsion. He was seen by a local doctor who found his well and advised the family to see a paediatrician at home. In the past he had an afebrile fit at the age of 3 years and had been well since

Yours sincerely...

Your task is to take a focused history and discuss the management plan with him and his parents

You have 13 minutes to take the history. There will be a warning bell at 9 min and at 13 minutes Robin and his parents will leave the room. You will have another 9 min to discuss the management plan with parents. (AG)

Focused history taking:
• Introduce yourself to patient and his parents.
• Thanks for coming and clarify the role and concerns.
• Engage Julian asking him if he knows why he has come to the hospital?
• Get parents to narrate the problem in their words.

Do not open with:
• Details of birth history
• Immunization history

Suggested Guide

Convulsions are a common clinical problem and candidates in the examination are given realistic scenarios.

While waiting outside the station draw up a mental scheme of how you would like to run the 'consultation'. Follow the structure that you would normally have for such a clinical problem. Remember this is as much a test of your communication skills as of you being systematic in gathering information about a specific aspect of the patient's illness. Also remember active listening – two ears and one mouth – use in the same proportion.

First introduce yourself to the parents and the Julian. Clarify the reasons for attending the clinic and your role.
• Engage Julian in an age appropriate conversation and can ask him if he knows why he has come to the hospital? You can continue with what he did in the morning, etc. Then you can say that 'is it Ok to ask Mummy if she knows?"

It is important to start with the details of presenting complaints: Convulsions in this case: Try and lead with open questions

- What happened? Active listening, make mental notes, do not interrupt.
  - Clarify points
    - what was he doing just before?
      - did he knock/hurt himself?
    - was there general shaking of arms and legs or not?
    - what was his colour?
      - was he flushed and red, started fitting and then went blue?
      - was he pale and blue and then started fitting?
    - how long did it last?
    - was there a 'post-ictal period'?
    - after how long 'he came round'?

Repeat to parents what you have understood and give opportunity to clarify any points further.

You proceed:

- Past medical history and details of the previous convulsion
- Medications
- Birth history and significant illness should be checked, i.e. meningitis, trauma
- Systems review
- Family details, parents, siblings, their age and health
- Social and school activity, i.e. normal or special school, any concerns at school

Repeat the history to parents again and ask "Is there anything else you would like to tell me that you feel is important?"

At the end of the 8 minutes you should have **a family portrait**. What happened to Julian, any precipitating factors, associate past medical history, family history, how his illness is affecting family members (very anxious at present).

You should also have developed a management plan to discuss with family if asked or definitely with the examiner.

The plan could be:

- Initial explanation of a seizure.

Seizure or a convulsion happen when there is abnormal brain activity. And it can be due to 'faulty workings' in our brain or our heart as the brain needs a constant supply of oxygen and glucose and any interruption causes the brain to 'shut down' like a computer.

Our body and brain work on tiny amounts of electrical current that allows us to think, move our arms when we want or talk. The electrical activity in the brain is 'organized / regulated' allowing us to function normally. When the 'fit' comes from the brain—In some individuals at times the activity can go 'haywire and abnormal' causing the person to lose consciousness, fall to the ground and have abnormal jerky movements. They usually stop fitting within a few minutes but it can seem like ages.

If for some reason the heart stops working properly even for a short period, causing an interruption to the oxygen going to the brain, the brain computer just shuts down and the person will lose consciousness, fall to the ground and may have jerky movements. When flat on the ground, the blood flow normally resumes, the brain 'boots up' again and the person comes round gradually.

- To find the cause the following are usually needed/done:
  - Full blood count, electrolytes, calcium, magnesium, liver function tests
  - Event diary

  In case of seizure activity
  - 12 –lead ECG and/exercise test
  - EEG
  - Possible:
    - neuro imaging
    - 7-day event recorder – cardiac

  Further evaluation may be required by neurologists or cardiologists

A brief guide line for differential diagnosis for 'fits, faints or funny turns' and loss of consciousness/seizures – just to recap: all are not be applicable to Julian.

Neurological: Seizure disorders
- Generalized
  - Tonic—clonic: body stiffens, patient falls, Jerking
  - Tonic: muscle stiffen, sudden fall, rapid recovery
  - Atonic: brief loss of body tone - drop attack
  - Myoclonic: brief, sudden convulsion of part of or whole body
  - Absence (petit mal): Simple or complex associated with autonomic disturbances or automatisms.
  - Atypical absences
- Partial seizures: caused by electrical firing in one part of the brain.
- Complex partial seizure: most common form of epilepsy. Consciousness in impaired and often originates in the temporal lobe.
- Infantile spasms
- Migraine
- Benign paroxysmal vertigo

Cardiovascular:	Reflex anoxic seizure
	Vasovagal syncope ± seizure
	Prolonged QT syndrome
Metabolic:	Hypoglycaemia
	Hypocalcaemia—Di George syndrome
Respiratory:	Breath holding attacks
	Cough syncope
Drug overdose:	Tricyclic antidepressants
	Aerosol inhalation (unlikely at this age)

Other: Munchausen's by proxy

                         Infant masturbation

                         Non-Epileptic Attack Disorder: Pseudoseizures

Neonates: Jittery baby, brainstem release phenomenon

It is also definitely worth knowing and mentioning:
- Pharmacological drug treatment
- Implications on lifestyle
  - Swimming—always with a companion with adult supervision
  - Showers instead of baths and *not* to lock the bathroom
  - Cycling – use of helmet, normal precautions
  - Horse riding: use of helmet
  - Sleep: possibility of suffocation during a fit – hence no pillows for children
  - Travel: to take a copy of letter and list of medications from doctor
  - In older young people—driving and career choice.

HISTORY AND MANAGEMENT: CONSTIPATION AND ENCOPRESIS

Information given to the candidate

You are the registrar (candidate) in the clinic and are given this written information outside the station. You have up to 4 minutes to prepare and may want to note down your planned approach (*The examiner does not see this written plan.*)

Dear Doctor**Re: Gabriel Bradford, DOB 23/11/2004**Gabriel is a 8-year-old girl whose parents are very concerned about her soiling and tendency to hide dirty knickers in her wardrobe. We have tried laxatives such as lactulose and senna with no benefit. Thank you for you advice.Y.S.*Dr Smith* **You are requested to take a focussed history and answer any queries parents may have. Discuss with the examiner your history and management plan later.You do not have to examine Gabriel.**

You have 13 minutes to complete the history taking; a warning bell will be given at the end 9 minutes. The last 9 minutes will be your discussion with the examiner and the patient will not be present (SP/AG).

A suggested approach to discuss with the family
Introduce yourself to the family and clarify the agenda for the consultation.

Speak to Gabriel first and involve her in the discussion. Use age appropriate language.

While speaking to parents you may follow scheme.

Presenting complaints
• Frequency of bowel opening
• Stool consistency
• Pain/difficulty in passing stools
• Soiling – how often
• Medications being used now and previously
• Dietary details

Past medical history:
• How and when parents first noticed this as a problem
• What all has been tried
• Passage of meconium—if delayed consider CF, Hirschsprung, hypothyroid, etc.

Social history:
• Parents and siblings.
• When were siblings continent or did they have similar problems
• Parents attitude to the 'disability'.

- How is the family coping with the problem.
  - Any traumatic experience in the family
  - Health of other siblings in family – chronic illness
  - Death of a grand parent
  - Divorce or separation of parents
  - Death of a pet
  - Change of school or issues about bullying
  - Strategies used by them for toilet training

Management strategies: The most important information to discuss with parents is that constipation is a very common problem. They are not alone and with help things will improve.
 It will be important to:
- Manage medication,
- Diet
- Behaviour as they are all closely interlinked.

Discussion with the examiner (a suggested scheme that may follow)
- There will be active interaction with the examiner during these 9 minutes
- Remember he has been listening to you take the history.
- Summarising your relevant history and important negatives.
- An approach to managing constipation (please see notes below)
- Disability caused to the child
- Medical and non-medical approach may be necessary at the same time
- Age appropriate counselling may need mentioning
- Involvement of the continence nurse

NOTE

Constipation with Soiling

It is a very common problem that causes great social difficulties for the child and family.

 Usually children have control over their bowels by the age of four, though some children naturally take longer. An occasional accident is nothing to worry about. Children generally become aware of the social stigma attached to soiling themselves.

 Generally constipation starts early on in infancy. Quite often following a transient viral illness, due to decreased fluid intake during the illness the stools become harder than usual and the child finds it uncomfortable to defecate. This leads to period of 'holding' on to the stools till such time when they pass a large bulky stool, usually quite firm. This causes discomfort and quite often an anal fissure that cause mild blood staining of stools and intense pain. This leads to further reluctance to pass stools.

At times of passing stools the child looks as straining very hard to pass stools with flushed face. However, he/she is trying to tightly close the anal sphincter so as *not* to pass stools at that time to avoid the pain Body physiology being what it is – stools cannot be held on for ever. A stage comes when some stools will leak through leading to unpleasant smells that stigmatize the child leading to embarrassment, low esteem and anxiety.

Another side effect of holding on to stools is that a hard mass forms in the rectum. This causes persistent dilatation of the internal sphincter thus leading to a loss of the 'feeling of urge' to defecate. The large bulk of stool becomes difficult to pass and as a result loose stools leak around it cause 'constant' soiling.

The child is usually quite embarrassed and often bullied by his peers and often misunderstood by his parents as being 'lazy' in not going to the toilet appropriately. This leads him to passing stools and hiding the evidence – dirty under pants – making matters worse.

The stool types have been 'standardised' for their consistency and 'Paediatric Bristol stool chart' is commonly used that differentiates stools in 7 categories. Rabbit dropping' (type 1) to gravy (type 7) (*see* page 190 for the stool chart).

Management Strategies

The most important information to discuss with parents is that constipation is a very common problem. They are not alone and with help things will improve.

It will be important to:
- Manage medication,
- Diet
- Behaviour as they are all closely interlinked.

Explain the mechanism of how the child has got so far as described above— from normal regular stools to irregular hard tools to soiling and then being disabled by it due to social pressures and self embarrassment.

The further plan needs to be discussed and agreed: Initial disimpaction
- Empty the colon
- Make the stools so soft so as to pass without discomfort
- Establish regular bowel habit pattern
- Suggest sitting on the toilet for 5–10 minutes at set time
  This 'long' time is needed so child can 'disconnect mentally' from the activity he/she was engaged with and can concentrate on passing stools'. It is important to have this time when the family schedule is not rushed and there are not lots of other activities happening.
- Keep a diary of stools so progress can be reviewed and encouraged.

The usual treatment plan should be to keep the stools soft and being able to pass without any discomfort for a period of a few weeks till the child 'forget' the trauma of passing stools and it become a regular daily activity. The stools can then be 'hardened' to normal consistency so as not to cause any discomfort by decreasing the medication.

Initial disimpaction can be:
- Enema under mild sedation
- Increasing dosage of Movicol® laxative
- In some case disempaction by paediatric surgeons.

The common type of laxatives are:
- Bulking agents: Lactulose
- Stimualants: Senna; Picosulphate
- Softner + bulk: Polyglycols–Movicol

A strategy used by me in cases with severe over loading of colon palpable per abdomen (avoid doing rectal examination in children as far as possible):
- Discuss plan with parents and have their acceptance
- Admit the child to day ward for an enema under light sedation: nasal midazolam. This has the advantage of child not remembering the comparatively unpleasant procedure of enema, relaxes them and allows large bulky stools to pass and is quick compared to the oral regime of disimpaction, it is recommended by some to use increasing doses of Movicol that can take up to two weeks or longer.

Parents and staff are generally amazed at the size and amount of stools the child passes.
- Commence the child on Movicol: 2–3 sachets per day, can be taken over 12 hours in their favourite drink—this to prevent the stools form hardening again. The amount of Movicol can be increased if required and this should be explained to parents.
- Child may initially pass stools in pull up pants/nappies till they are confident to use toilet.
- Advised to set regular time aside to go and sit on the toilet and try to pass stools.
- A hole can be cut in the pull up pants/nappy while sitting on toilet to build confidence.

Review the child at regular intervals, more frequently initially and also encouraging more fibre in the diet.

It can be useful to offer a reward for not soiling, for example, a sticker chart for when they are keeping their pants clean. However, do keep in mind that more often the child is not in control of his bowels and this may lead to frustration. Encourage the positive and do not make the negative a deemed punishment.

It is also important to address and acknowledge the psychological stress the child is feeling and often not able to communicate effectively.

Counselling should be provided when ever possible.

It may be necessary to liaise with school to allow the treatment regime to work.

I personally realised quite late in my career how big disability constipation and soiling are to the child and affect the whole family. The social life is greatly disturbed as they cannot go out as the child 'smells', difficult for child to participate in normal activities like 'sleep over', the child generally feels bloated, eats poorly due to constant abdominal discomfort and may not be quite as active as his peers. These things are only realized retrospectively when the treatment has been effective. The number of parents who have later said that they feel their child is a different person, eating better, being more active and lively.

In my opinion, treating constipation, soiling and encopresis well is worthwhile.

Paediatric Bristol Stool Chart is an important tool while eliciting a history of constipation. Concept by Professor DCA Candy and Emma Davey, based on the Bristol Stool Form Scale produced by Dr K W Heaton, Reader in Medicine at the University of Bristol. 2000 Norgine Pharmaceuticals Ltd.

It will be useful to go through the NICE guideline on childhood constipation as well. http://www.nice.org.uk/CG99

HISTORY TAKING AND MANAGEMENT PLANNING: ENURESIS

Information given to the candidate

You are the registrar (candidate) in the clinic and are given this written information outside the station. You have up to 4 minutes to prepare and may want to note down your planned approach. (*The examiner does not see this written plan.*)

Dear Doctor

Thank you for seeing Robin. He is a 12-year-old boy and has been bed wetting. He is the only child. Both his parents are teachers and are very anxious.
We checked his urine and it was clear.
Yours sincerely
GP

Your task is to take a focused history and discuss the management plan with him and his parents if they wish. You will later discuss with the examiner.

You do not have to examine Robin

You have 13 minutes to take the history. There will be a warning bell at 9 minutes and at 13 minutes Robin and his parents will leave the room. You will have another 9 minutes. to discuss the management plan with examiner. (UP/AG)

Focused history taking

- Introduce yourself to patient and his parents.
- Thanks for coming and clarify the role and concerns.
- Acknowledge letter from GP and ask open question to Robin asking him to narrate the problem.
  - How is it affecting him
  - What he finds most difficult
  - How are daytime symptoms
- Involve parents next to fill in any additional information
  - find out if he was completely dry at any time of his life
  - differentiate primary or secondary enuresis
  - when he was potty trained.
  - has he any daytime symptom.
  - does he sleep through night
  - does he have one big patch or multiple small wet patches throughout the night.
  - is the toilet he readily accessible to him.
- Drinking habit including daytime drinking amount and last drink before bedtime.

- Does he have lots of fizzy drink, caffeinated drinks.
- Is he constipated.
- Stress at school
- Any psychological precipitating factor ie family difficulties, deaths, etc.
- Explore positive family history
  - age when parents dry
- What treatment options that have been tried
- **Conclude with a summary to the patient and ask that if there is anything else they would like to add you have not asked.**

You should then discuss your management plan with examiner:
- Common problem
- Explain how normal bladder control is acquired and works
- Assure—as *no* daytime concerns – 'connections' are right between brain and bladder.
- Offer to discuss various strategies
- Keep the language simple

Do not ask
- Details of birth history
- Immunization history

What is expected from the candidate?

Introduce yourself to the patient and family.
- Focused open questions
- Establish diagnosis between primary (never been dry for >6 months) or secondary enuresis.
- Differentiate between small bladder capacity versus suboptimal ADH secretion or both.
- Explore family history, family dynamic, accessibility to toilet, emotional and psychological aspects
- Able to summarise and discuss differential diagnosis.
- Able to discuss the management plan options including:
  - increased daytime drinking,
  - avoid constipation,
  - modification of lifestyle,
  - alarm pad,
  - specific medication
    - detrusor stabilising agent
    - desmotab – desmopressin (ADH).

It will be useful to update yourself with NICE guidelines. http://www.nice.org.uk/nicemedia/pdf/CG54NICEguideline.pdf

HISTORY TAKING AND MANAGEMENT PLANNING: ASTHMA WITH POOR GROWTH

Information given to the candidate
You are the registrar (candidate) in the clinic and are given this written information outside the station. You have up to 4 minutes to prepare and may want to note down your planned approach.
(*The examiner does not see this written plan.*)

Role: You are the Specialist Registrar

Setting: Children's Outpatients Clinic at District General Hospital

You are talking to: Gregory a 6-year-old boy and his mother

Task: Take a focused history, aiming to explore the problem indicated as you would in the clinical situation. You may answer questions that the subject (role player) may pose to you. After the consultation the examiner will focus on your management planning.

Dear Dr..........

Re: Gregory D age 8 years

Gregory has been seen regularly at your outpatient clinic mainly because of respiratory problems. His mother has noted Gregory to have become tired and listless over the past 3 months. On examination I can find no significant abnormalities.

I should be very grateful if you would see him and advise on appropriate investigations and management.

Yours sincerely,
Dr G. Smith
General Practitioner

Background information: Gregory has been seen regularly at the Outpatient Clinic, having asthma and eczema.

Any other information: The current findings on physical examination are that Gregory is thin (0.4th centile) and short (2nd centile) but is otherwise normal.

Your task is to take a focused history and discuss the management plan with him and his parents if they wish. You will later discuss with the examiner.

You do not have to examine Gregory.

You have 13 minutes to take the history. There will be a warning bell at 9 minutes and at 13 minutes Robin and his parents will leave the room. You will have another 9 minutes to discuss the management plan with examiner.
(AG/SE)

Focused history taking

- Introduces self and greets both parent and the child
- Asks how Gregory has been doing.
  - Start with information given in GP's letter and confirms the information
- Asks a open question about the current concerns in relation to medical information given in GP letter.
- Listen to the concerns without disturbing but can ask closed questions to clarify.
- Concerns in this case was poor growth.
  - Asks diet history and ask about food allergies
  - Asks about acute episodes of asthma needing admissions and interval symptoms. Ask about medications-steroids, reliever and preventer medications
- Eczema—assess the severity and medications
- Food allergies—which food and what allergic reactions, how the diagnosis made-skin prick tests
- Perinatal history about milk allergy
- Family history of asthma, eczema, food allergies
- Growth and development—ask for the red book
- Ask about input by asthma nurse and dietician
- Ask the best peak flow and diary with daily peak flow readings.
- Immunisation: routine and flu jab and swine flu jab.
- Ask whether he has epipen at home and school
- Allergy bracelet
- Addresses the concerns—could be issues related to bullying at school!!
- Poor growth
- Poorly controlled asthma
- Poorly controlled eczema
- What treatment options that have been tried.
- **Conclude with a summary to the patient and ask that if there is anything else they would like to add, you have not asked.** You should then be ready to discuss your management.

Role Player Information

As the role player will be the parent of a "real" child, there is no need to provide them with written background details in advance of the examination. The Host Examiner should brief the parent on what to expect and on what information to volunteer to the candidates and how to uniformly "perform".

It will be useful to update yourself with NICE and SIGN guidelines.

Video Section

We cannot provide video clips in the book.

To give some semblance we have given more than one photograph to a clinical scenario.

Details and video clips will be available on related website www.mrcpchclinicals.org.

The information in the following pictures/videos is confidential and privileged. You are expected to follow your Medical Council guidelines on Patient confidentiality. By continuing to participate you accept your responsibility.

There will be a short statement leading into the pictures/video. This will be followed by one or more questions. Each question will have a stem followed by a number of options. Please mark as per instructions. If there are no specific instructions – mark each option as true/false.

To get maximum benefit–do not jump to the answer. See the image carefully, write down what you observe, differential diagnosis and then attempt the question. Later read about the subject as these are common scenarios.

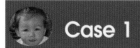

A 3-day-old baby born by assisted instrumental delivery is noted to have a progressive swelling of the right side of his head.

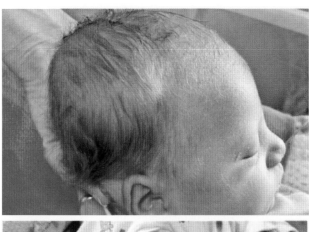

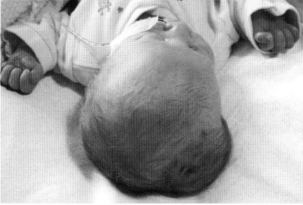

Q. The most appropriate management is:
  A. Blood transfusion
  B. Check bilirubin
  C. Inform parents child is likely to suffer brain damage
  D. Skull X-ray
  E. Ultrasound scan of head

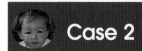

A 2-month-old infant presented with febrile illness. He had a pure growth of *E. coli* from the urine. Investigations showed the following

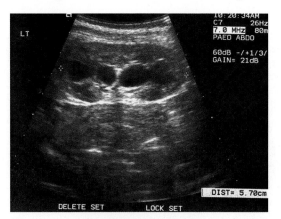

Renal ultrasound scan

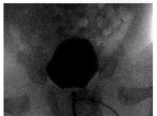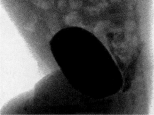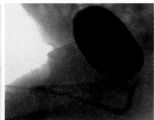

Micturating cystourethrogram

Q. All of the following are correct except: (choose 1)
   A. Co-amoxiclav is the first line antimicrobial
   B. High risk of PUJ (pelvi-ureteric junction) obstruction
   C. Refer to paediatric urologist
   D. Shows grade four reflux
   E. Urgent catheterization

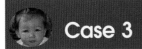
A 3-month-old Alfie is brought to hospital by his parents. They give history of excessive crying for the past 3 days and no history of trauma. Initial investigations show normal blood count. X-rays show:

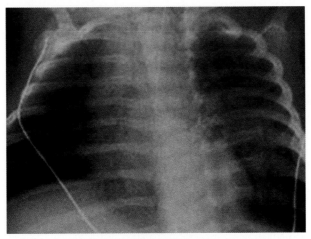

Chest X-ray

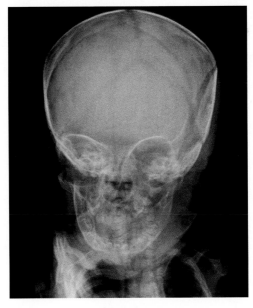

Skull X-ray

Q1: The next most appropriate action will be:
   A. Arrange for Alfie to be taken in care
   B. Full skeletal survery
   C. Fundoscopy
   D. Refer to social service
   E. Test for osteogensis imperfecta

Q2: The X-rays/radiographs show: (choose two)
   A. Craniosynostosis
   B. Dextrocardia
   C. Injuries occurred at birth
   D. Injuries occurred at different times
   E. Injuries occurred at same time
   F. Left skull fracture
   G. Pneumomediastinum
   H. Right pneumothorax
   I. Right skull fracture

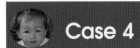

John, a 10-year-old boy has been referred by the school nurse for his bruises. He gives history of falling and hurting himself in the playground. You note the following during your examination.

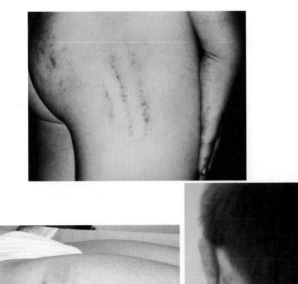

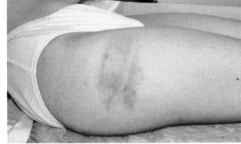

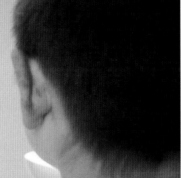

Q. What will be the next most appropriate action?
   A. Arrange for John to be taken in care
   B. Ring the school nurse to inform that bruises are compatible with history
   C. Skeletal survey
   D. Refer to ophthalmology for fundoscopy
   E. Refer to social service

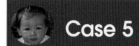

This 2-year-old girl has been referred by her General Practitioner. Her mother is concerned about her abnormal physical development. She is otherwise reported to be achieving milestones normally.

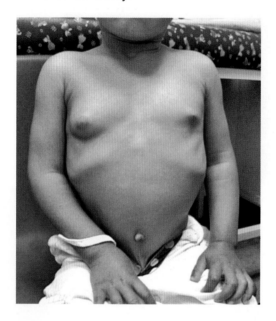

Q. What will be the next two most appropriate management in this child?
  A. Bone age
  B. Check blood glucose
  C. Check electrolytes
  D. Chromosomal analysis
  E. CT scan head
  F. LH/FSH ratio
  G. MRI brain
  H. Reassure mother and arrange follow up in 1 year,
  I. Urinary steroid profile

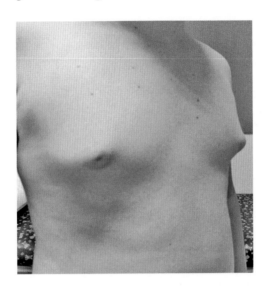

Tom, a 13-year-old boy is referred by his GP due to concerns about bullying at school. He is shy to go swimming.

Q. The following will be appropriate:
   A. Bone age
   B. Chromosome analysis
   C. Explain it is physiological and arrange for follow-up.
   D. Refer to a plastic surgeon
   E. Unlikely to regress spontaneously

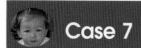

Tom, a 1-month-old baby is seen in a multidisciplinary clinic.

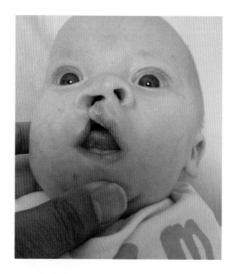

Q. His parents need not be concerned about:
   A. Developmental delay
   B. Feeding difficulty
   C. Glue ear
   D. Hearing problems
   E. Speech problems

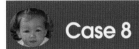

Elizabeth is a 5-day-old baby. She has poor feeding and demonstrates:

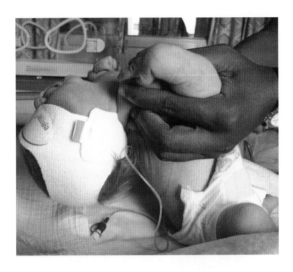

Q. This is unlikely to be due to: (choose one)
  A. Neonatal myoclonus
  B. Overwhelming sepsis
  C. Prader-Willi syndrome
  D. Severe birth asphyxia
  E. Spinal muscular atrophy (Werdnig-Hoffmann disease)

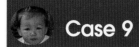

A 4-week-old baby, born to Caucasian parents is reviewed for failure to gain weight. You note:

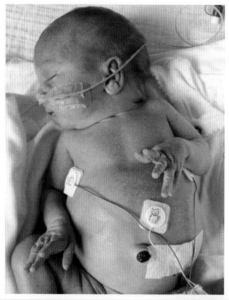

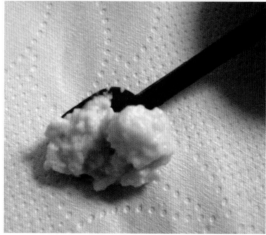

Q1. The following need not be considered in the diagnosis:
   A. Biliary atresia
   B. Breast milk jaundice
   C. CMV infection
   D. Hypothyroidism
   E. Toxoplasmosis

Q2. Which of the following two investigations should be organised next:
   A. Abdominal ultrasound scan
   B. Alkaline phosphatase
   C. Bilirubin
   D. Bilirubin total/direct (unconjugated: conjugated)
   E. Blood group
   F. Coomb's test
   G. Haemoglobin
   H. HIDA scan (hepatoiminodiacetic acid)
   I. Lymphocyte count

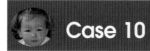

A 12-year-old boy presents with febrile episodes for 2 weeks.

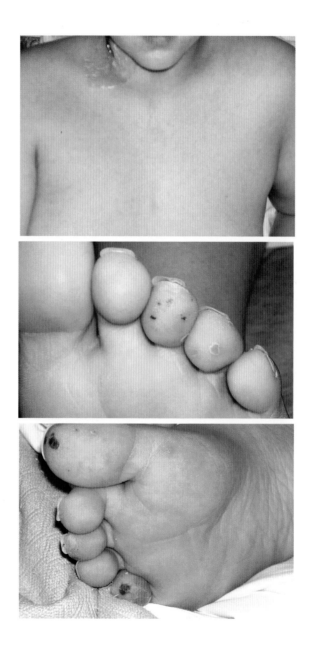

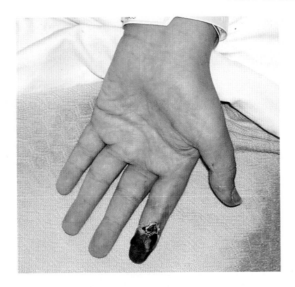

Q. The following two will be the next appropriate management steps:
   A. Blood cultures when pyrexial
   B. CXR
   C. ECG
   D. Echocardiogram
   E. Full blood count
   F. Gentamicin IV
   G. Liver function test
   H. Penicillin IV
   I. Sleeping heart rate

An 18-month-old girl is admitted with 3 month history of being progressively lethargic.

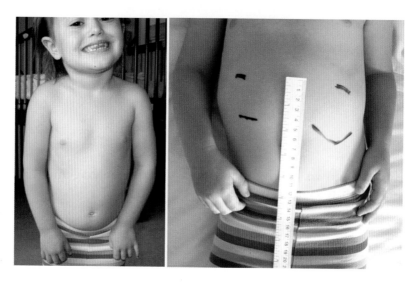

Her FBC shows:
Hb 6.9 gm%
WBC 37.8 × 10⁹/L
Neutrophils 5.7 × 10⁹/L
Lymphocytes 27.4 × 10⁹/L
Monocytes 3.9 × 10⁹/L
Eosinophils 0.2 × 10⁹/L
Platelets 445 × 10⁹/L
Reticulocytes 499

Q. What will be next best management option:
    A. Bone marrow aspirate
    B. Immunoglobilins IV
    C. Monospot test
    D. Parvovirus serology
    E. Steroids IV

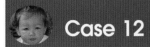

A 1-year-old boy is admitted with respiratory distress. Loud pan systolic murmur, 3/6 Lower left sternal border. Liver 3 cm enlarged.

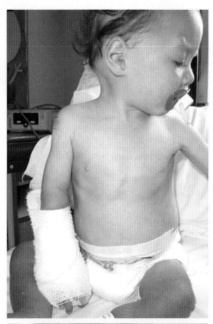

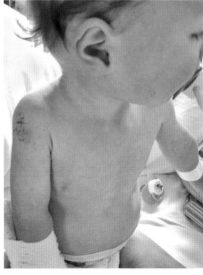

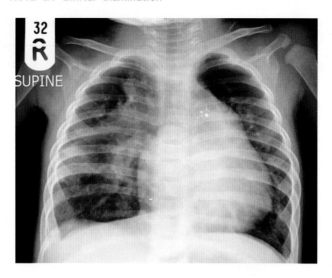

Q. The next most appropriate management is:
   A. Arrange removal of foreign bodies
   B. Fluids 180 ml/ kg /day
   C. Frusemide 20 mg IV
   D. Hydrocortisone IV
   E. Salbutamol nebulised

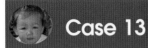

Three and a half year old boy is admitted to the ward for observations.

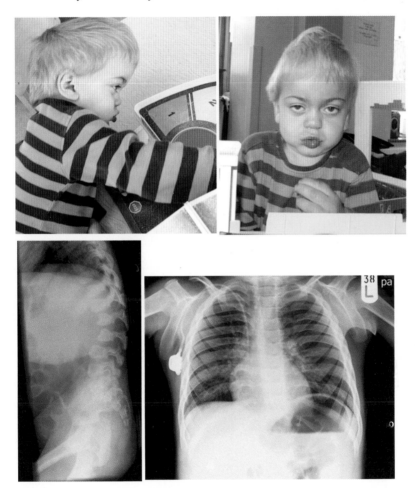

Q1. Hematopoietic stem cell transplantation (HSCT) in children under 2 years does not improve:
A. Corneal clouding
B. Facial coarseness
C. Hearing loss
D. Hepatosplenomegaly
E. Survival

Q2. Enzyme replacement therapy with Laronidase does not improve:
- A. Cognitive function
- B. Growth
- C. Hepatomegaly
- D. Joint mobility
- E. Sleep apnoea

A 5-year-old girl is seen in the clinic for abdominal pain and bilious vomiting off and on for 4 months. She was operated in the neonatal period.

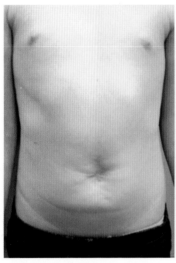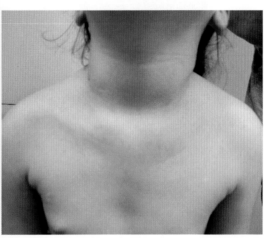

Q. She is likely to be suffering from:
   A. Constipation
   B. Intussusceptions
   C. Intestinal obstruction
   D. Migraine
   E. Urinary tract infection

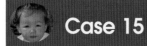

A new born baby is noted to have ambiguous genitalia and is very pale

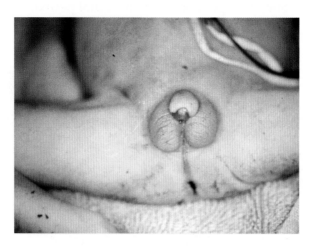

Q1. What is next management: (choose 1)
 A. 10% dextrose – saline bolus
 B. Chromosome analysis
 C. Group and cross match blood
 D. Transfuse O –ve blood
 E. Urinary steroid profile

Q2. After initial resuscitation and blood transfusion the following are necessary for management except:
 A. Chromosome analysis
 B. Electrolytes
 C. Laparotomy for gonadal identification
 D. Ultrasound scan of abdomen
 E. Urinary steroid profile

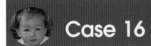

A 1-month-old is admitted with poor feeding, vomiting and abnormal movements. On examination she is noted to have Heart rate 180/min, Respiration: 60/min, CRT 4 sec:

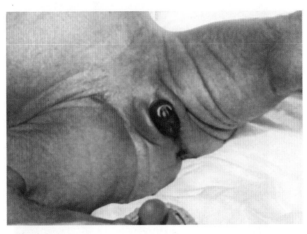

Q1. The following two investigations should be done next to help with underlying diagnosis:
   A. 17 OH progesterone
   B. Calcium
   C. Creatinine
   D. Electrolytes
   E. Full blood count
   F. Hydrocortisone
   G. Magnesium
   H. Renin
   I. Urea/creatinine ratio

Q2. The following will be appropriate next management: choose 1
   A. 0.4% NaCl solution bolus a 20 ml/kg
   B. 0.9% NaCl bolus 10 ml /kg
   C. 0.9% NaCl bolus 20 ml/kg
   D. 3.0% Saline infusion
   E. 50% Dextrose bolus

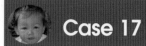

A 2-year-old girl is referred by her GP. Her mother is concerned about her facial appearance.

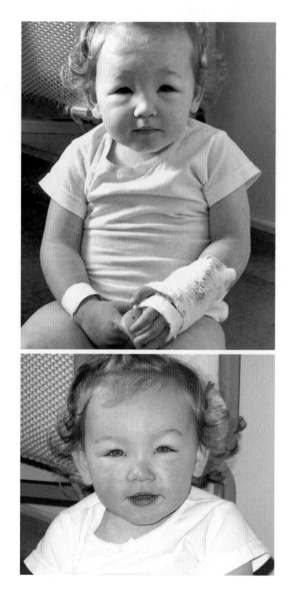

Q1. The following blood investigations should be done next: (choose 4)
A. Albumin
B. Cholesterol
C. Complement
D. Gamma globulin sub class
E. Haemoglobin

Q2. Her urine shows 4 + albuminurea. Further management will include: (choose 4)
A. Daily weight
B. Fluid restriction
C. Penicillin
D. Prednisolone
E. Renal biopsy

A 6-month-old boy is reviewed for faltering growth, poor feeding and dusky episodes following review by his health visitor.

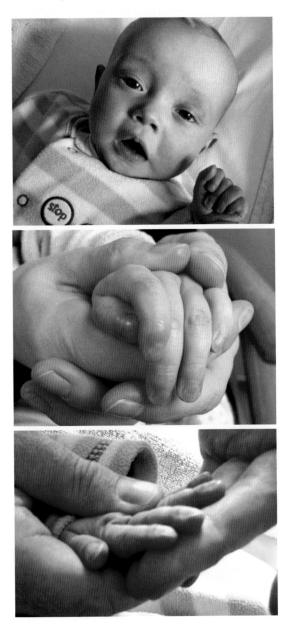

Q. The following will be next in management:
   A. Capillary blood gases
   B. Lung functions
   C. Pulse oximetry
   D. Sweat test
   E. Urea and electrolytes

A 4-month-old baby girl is admitted with history of nappy rash for 3 months and rash round her mouth for 2 months not improving with topical treatment.

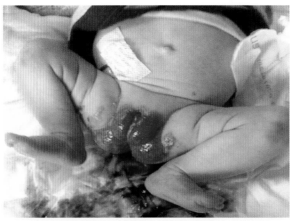

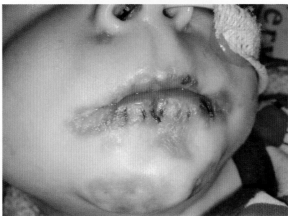

Q1. The following investigation should be done next to assist with diagnosis. Assay of serum:

A. Copper

B. Iron

C. Magnesium

D. Selenium

E. Zinc

Q2. The following feed will be most appropriate for the infant:
   A. Amino acid formula milk
   B. Anti-reflux milk formula
   C. High calorie infant formula
   D. Modified cow's milk formula
   E. Partially hydrolysed formula

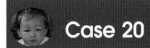

A 20-month-old girl is admitted with initial vesicular rash and recent 4-day history of high fever.

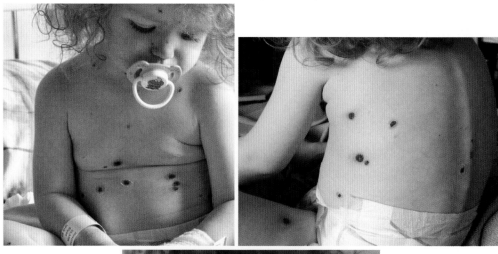

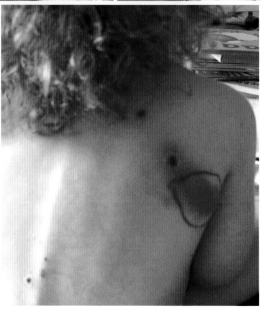

Q1. The following is indicated as appropriate next line of management:
   A. Blood culture
   B. Complement assessment
   C. Serum immunoglobulins sub-types
   D. T cell function
   E. Viral culture

Q2. The following treatment is indicated:
   A. Acyclovir
   B. Immunoglobulin
   C. Penicillin + Flucloxacillin IV
   D. Penicillin + Gentamicin IV
   E. Penicillin IV

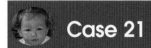

John an ex-premature baby, born at 30 weeks presents with URTI symptoms for 3 days.

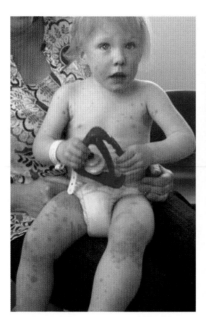 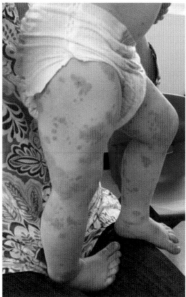

Q. What will be the most appropriate next step:
   A. Amoxicillin
   B. ASO titre
   C. Chlorpheniramine maleate
   D. Hydrocortisone
   E. Mycoplasma serology

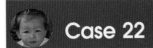

A term male infant has umbilical lines inserted and is in headbox oxygen with
FiO_2 0.4 (40%)

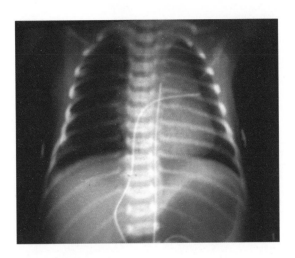

**Q. The following blood results are compatible with a sample from the UVC.
(Choose 2 answers)**
A. pCO_2 3.0 kPa
B. pCO_2 7.0 kPa
C. pCO_2 8.5 kPa
D. pH: 7.10
E. pO_2 3.0 kPa
F. pO_2 10.5 kPa
G. pO_2 4.0 kPa

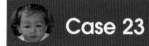

Newborn baby noted to have dysmorphic features and feeding difficulty.

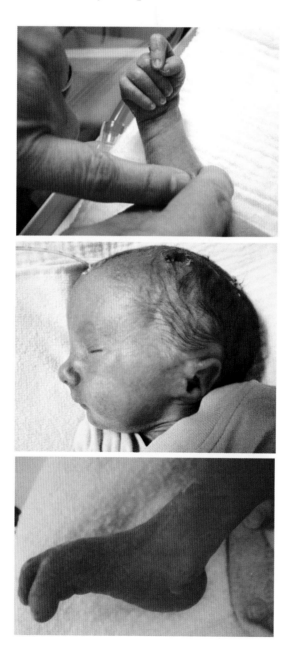

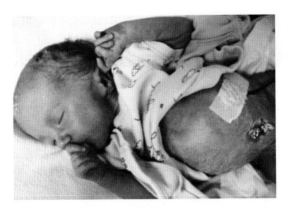

Q. What chromosome pattern would be most likely?
   A. Deletion 6p
   B. Deletion 9p4q
   C. Trisomy 13
   D. Trisomy 18
   E. Trisomy 21

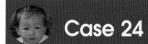

A newborn baby is noted to have severe respiratory distress following birth. CXRs are:

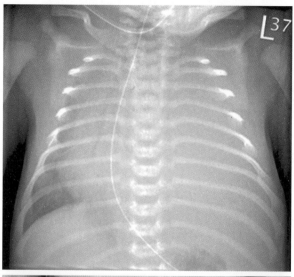

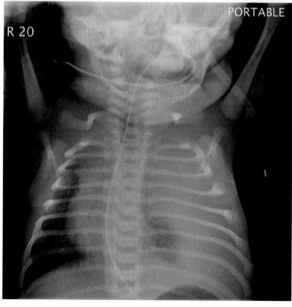

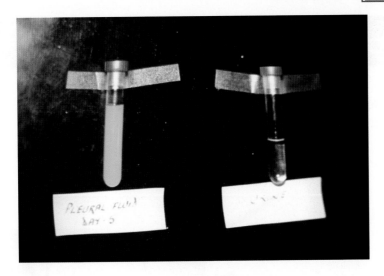

Q. **What will be the management for this newborn**
  A. 10% dextrose
  B. Hydrolysed formula feeds
  C. Normal milk feeds
  D. TPN for 2 days followed by milk
  E. TPN for 3–4 weeks

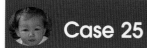

A 8-year-old deteriorated during hospital admission over 3 hours with rapidly progressing nonblanching rash.

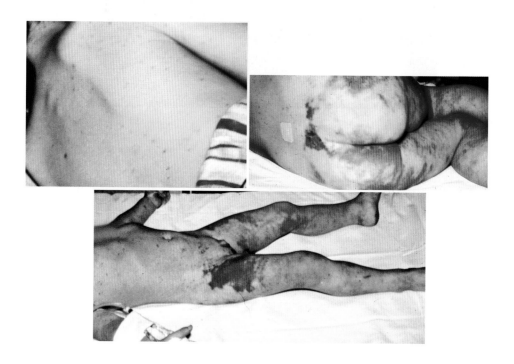

Q. It is safe to give fluid resuscitation with:
A. 0.9% Normal saline + 10% Dextrose 80 ml /kg
B. 0.9% Normal saline + 5% Dextrose 100 ml / kg
C. 0.9% Normal saline 150 ml/kg bolus
D. 0.9% Normal saline 40 ml/kg bolus
E. 0.9% Normal saline 80 ml/kg bolus

ANSWERS TO VIDEO SECTION

Case 1

Answer (B) Check bilirubin.
Cephalhaematoma develops over the first few days. It regresses spontaneously and does not need any specific treatment in most cases. It may contribute to high bilirubin load.

Case 2

Answer (B) High risk of PUJ obstruction.
Renal ultrasound scan shows evidence of hydronephrosis with dilated collecting system.
MCUG shows large bladder with narrowing at outlet – posterior urethral valves.
The obstruction is at bladder neck. This can also leads to prune-belly syndrome.

Case 3

Q1: Answer (D) Refer to social service.
There are multiple injuries not compatible with the history provided.
Callus formation noted on ribs is indicative of an injury at least 2 weeks old.
Q2: Answers (D) Injuries occurred at different times (F) left skull fracture
Chest X-ray show multiple left rib fractures with callus formation.
Skull X-ray shows fracture in the left temporal parietal area.

Case 4

Answer (E) Refer to social services.
Multiple bruises of different colour shades suggest different age. Also straight lines on the thigh are likely to be finger marks.
Injuries to the pinna are also highly suggestive of NAI.
(*see* body map).

Case 5

Answer: (H) Reassure mother and arrange follow up in 1 year, (I) Urinary steroid profile

pediatrics.uchicago.edu/chiefs/documents/**Precocious**Puberty-Brian.pdf

Case 6

Answer (C) Explain it is physiological and arrange for follow up.

- Gynaecomastia is the most common reason for male breast evaluation. The condition is common in infancy and adolescence, as well as in middle-aged to older adult males. It is estimated that 60–90% of infants have transient gynaecomastia due to the high estrogen state of pregnancy.
- The next peak is seen during puberty, with a prevalence ranging from 4–69%. Some reports have shown a transient increase in oestradiol concentration at the onset of puberty in boys who develop gynaecomastia. Pubertal gynaecomastia usually has an onset in boys aged 10–12 years. It generally regresses within 18 months, and persistence is uncommon in men older than 17 years.

  Ref: http://emedicine.medscape.com/article/120858-overview

Case 7

Answer (A) Developmental delay

- Midline cleft palates are associated with chromosomal abnormalities
- Repair of cleft lip occurs in first few months: palate within 18 months
- Coordinated management by multidisciplinary team is recommended

Ref: http://www.cdc.gov/ncbddd/birthdefects/CleftLip.html

Case 8

Answer (A) Neonatal myoclonus

- Important to distinguish between Central and peripheral hypotonia
- Over whelming sepsis can cause temporary hypotonia
- Infants may be categorised by careful history and examination

Ref
http://pedsinreview.aappublications.org/cgi/content/abstract/6/8/237
Pediatrics in Review. 1985;6:237–243. doi:10.1542/pir.6-8-237)
© 1985 American Academy of Pediatrics
http://web.squ.edu.om/med-Lib/MED CD/E CDs/
CHILD%20NEUROLOGY/docs/ch81.pdf

Case 9

Q1: Answer (B) Breast milk jaundice.

Q2: Answer (A) Abdominal ultrasound scan, (D) Bilirubin total/direct
(unconjugated: conjugated)

- Obstructive jaundice is important to identify early as surgery is recommended by 3 months

Ref: http://emedicine.medscape.com/article/974786

Case 10

Answer (A) Blood cultures when pyrexial, (D) Echocardiogram
- Features are due to bacteremia, local cardiac invasion by organisms, embolization
- Turbulent flow damages the endothelium to which platelets and fibrin can adhere
- Most common organism *Streptococcus viridans, Staphylococcus aureus*
- Culture negative endocarditis

Ref: http://emedicine.medscape.com/article/896540-overview

Case 11

Answer (C) Monospot test (for EBV)
Ref: http://emedicine.medscape.com/article/963894

Case 12

Answer (C) Frusemide 20 mg IV

The respiratory distress is due to congestive heart failure.

The foreign bodies are:
1. PDA closure device
2. Ingested piece of metal

Case 13

Q1: Answer (A) Corneal clouding.
Q2: Answer (A) Cognitive function.

General note

Diagnosis is Mucopolysaccharidosis.

X-ray spine shows characterstic 'beaking' of the vertebrae. The ribs are flattened. Children are normal at birth and develop dysmorphic features during the early years.

Enzyme replacement is recommended for treatment of non-CNS manifestations.
- Progressive mental retardation and characteristic bone changes
- Organomegaly with cloudy cornea due to deposition
- Enzyme replacement therapy and Stem cell transplant are offered treatments.

Enzyme replacement therapy (ERT) with laronidase, is licensed for treatment of the non-CNS manifestations of MPS I. It improves liver size, linear growth, joint mobility, breathing, and sleep apnoea in persons with attenuated disease. The timing of the initiation of ERT is likely to influence the outcome.

Hematopoietic stem cell transplantation (HSCT) in selected children with severe MPS I before age two years can increase survival, reduce facial coarseness and hepatosplenomegaly, improve hearing, and maintain normal heart function. HSCT does not significantly improve skeletal manifestations or corneal clouding. HSCT may slow the course of cognitive decline in children with mild, but not significant, cognitive impairment at the time of transplantation.

Ref

http://www.ncbi.nlm.nih.gov/books/NBK1162/

http://ghr.nlm.nih.gov/condition/mucopolysaccharidosis-type-i

Case 14

Answer (C) Intestinal obstruction.

The obstruction is due to adhesions following surgery in the neonatal period.
- Absence of umbilicus
- Look for other scar marks from drains etc.
- Bilious vomiting is a significant sign in children

Note the abdominal scar with absent umbilicus. Closer inspection of neck upper chest shows scar mark in keeping with surgical insertion of central line. http://emedicine.medscape.com/article/975583-overview

Case 15

Q1: Answer (D) Transfuse O −ve blood

Q2: Answer (C) Laparotomy for gonadal indetification

Remember Resuscitation—Airway Breathing Circulation Disability/Drugs: Stabilising the newborn in the first objective – other management measures will follow.

http://www.mayoclinic.com/health/ambiguous-genitalia/DS00668/DSECTION=tests-and-diagnosis

http://www.nlm.nih.gov/medlineplus/ency/article/003269.htm

Case 16

Q1. Answer (A) 17 OH progesterone, (D) Electrolytes.
Q2. Answer (C) 0.9% NaCl bolus 20 ml/kg to rehydrate the infant.

Prominent clitoris should alert to inborn error of metabolism.

After samples are obtained to measure electrolyte, blood sugar, cortisol, aldosterone, and 17-hydroxyprogesterone concentrations, the patient should be treated with glucocorticoids based on suspected adrenal insufficiency. Treatment should not be withheld while confirmatory results are awaited because it may be life saving.

http://www.ncbi.nlm.nih.gov/pubmedhealth/PMH0001448/
http://www.nlm.nih.gov/medlineplus/ency/article/000411.htm
http://emedicine.medscape.com/article/919218-overview#a0104

Case 17

Q1: Answer (A, B, C, E)

- Working diagnosis is Nephrotic syndrome. Gamma globulin subclass are not the next line investigations.

Q2: Answer (A, B, C, D)

- Proteinuria, hypoalbuminemia, hypercholesterolemia.
- Minimal lesion commonest in children
- Trial of steroids first line without biopsy in discussion with tertiary unit.

Ref: http://emedicine.medscape.com/article/982920

Case 18

Answer (C) Pulse oximetry

It is important to establish that the child is cyanosed and the clinical signs evident are dusky appearance with clubbing

- Faltering growth—consider chronic disease
- Clubbing—cyanotic heart disease plus other causes.

Ref: http://www.ncbi.nlm.nih.gov/pmc/articles/PMC1777828/

Case 19

Q1. Answer (E) Zinc.

Acrodermatitis enteropathica. It cause resistant nappy rash and oral lesions.

Q2. Answer (A) Amino acid formula milk

The most easily absorbed formula as patient has 'enterocolitis' due to Zinc deficiency.

- Link lesions of various sites plus history
- Prolonged nonresponse to conventional treatment
- Learn various types of milk types: normal, partially hydrolysed, amino acid based.

Acrodermatitis enteropathica (AE) is an inborn error of zinc metabolism that is inherited as an autosomal recessive disorder. Symptoms in infancy typically include periorificial and acral dermatitis (see image below), diarrhoea, behavioral changes, and neurologic disturbances. In older children, faltering growth, anorexia, alopecia, nail dystrophy, and repeated infections are most common.

Zinc gluconate or sulfate is administered orally at a dosage of 1–3 mg/kg/d. Clinical response is observed within 5–10 days. Zinc gluconate or sulfate therapy is life-long for patients with AE.

Ref: http://emedicine.medscape.com/article/912075

Case 20

Q1: Answer (A) Blood culture

Secondary bacterial infection is the most likely cause and the first line investigation should be to identify the likely organism.

It is unlikely that child has immune deficiency and need not be looked for as first line investigations.

Q2: Answer (C) Penicillin + Flucloxacillin IV

Secondary bacterial infection—needs antibiotic cover. Infection is usually due to *Staphylococcus*. Hence Gentamicin is not indicated.
- Children seen admitted to hospital are only tip of an iceberg
- Secondary bacterial infection, with Gm +ve organisms can be fatal in chicken pox
- Infectivity + acyclovir – please read up

Ref: http://www.pediatricsdigest.mobi/content/108/5/e79.short

"Considerable morbidity with a comparatively high rate of encephalitis, osteomyelitis, and pyogenic arthritis. Although infectious complications were present in only 38.6% of the reported cases, they contributed disproportionately to the cases with chronic sequelae. Looking at these cases in more detail, *S pyogenes* involvement was identified as the major risk factor for invasive disease with an unfavorable long-term outcome. varicella-zoster virus, chickenpox/epidemiology, chickenpox/complications, encephalitis, cellulitis, osteomyelitis, necrotizing fasciitis, group A β-hemolytic streptococci, Europe."

Ref: Ziebold C, von Kries R, Lang R, Weigl J, Schmitt HJ. Severe complications of varicella in previously healthy children in Germany: a 1-year survey. *Pediatrics*. 2001 Nov;108(5):E79.

Case 21

Answer (C) Chlorpheniramine maleate
- Physical agents, drugs, foods and food additives, inhalants and infections may provoke urticaria.

Ref: http://www.nlm.nih.gov/medlineplus/ency/article/000845.htm
http://www.dermis.net/dermisroot/en/37185/diagnose.htm

Case 22

Answers (A) pCO_2 3.0 kPa, (F) pO_2 10.5 kPa

The key is that the UVC is sampling oxygenated blood returning from the lungs via the left pulmonary vein. The UVC has crossed across the foramen ovale into the left atrium.

Be sure of being able to differentiate umbilical venous and arterial catheters.

Case 23

Answer (D) Trisomy 18. (Edward syndrome)
- Second most common trisomy after trisomy 21.

Pictures show low set ears, single palmer crease, typical finger position and feet.

Management is essentially good communication with parents and supportive care.

Ref: http://emedicine.medscape.com/article/943463

Case 24

Answer (E) TPN for 3–4 weeks

Antenatal chylothorax presented with respiratory distress following birth. There is mediastinal shift evident by position of NGT in the chest. Fluid moved from the thorax to relieve distress initially. Subsequent management was TPN.

Chylothorax is more common in 'West' following surgery.

Ref:
http://www.uptodate.com/contents/diagnosis-and-management-of-chylothorax-and-cholesterol-effusions
http://cardiopedhnn.comfypage.com/site/UserFiles/Chylothorax.pdf

Case 25

Answer (D) 0.9% Normal saline 40 ml/kg bolus.

There is usually rapid deterioration with meningococcal sepsis. In this child it took only a few hours. Mortality is high but can be avoided with prompt and aggressive resuscitation and availability of intensive care.

The child will require more fluid but it is essential to secure the airway due to the risk of pulmonary oedema.
- Look up current guidelines
- Early respiratory and ionotropic support
- Prophylaxis for contacts

Ref: http://www.nlm.nih.gov/medlineplus/ency/article/001349.htm

Appendices

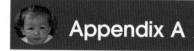

pGALS—A MUSCULOSKELETAL SCREENING ASSESSMENT FOR SCHOOL-AGED CHILDREN

The additions and amendments to the orignal adult GALS are highlighted in bold

SCREENING QUESTIONS

- Do you have any pain or stiffness in your joints, muscles or your back?
- Do you have any difficulty getting yourself dressed without any help?
- Do you have any difficulty going up and down stairs?

GAIT

- Observe the child walking
- "Walk on your tip-toes/walk on your heels"

ARMS

- "Put your hands out in front of you"
- "Turn your hands over and make a fist"
- "Pinch your index finger and thumb together"
- "Touch the tips of your fingers with your thumb"
- Squeeze the metacarpophalangeal joints
- "Put your hands together/put your hands back to back"
- "Reach up and touch the sky"
- "Look at the ceiling"
- "Put your hands behind your neck"

LEGS

- Feel for effusion at the knee
- "Bend and then straighten your knee" (active movement of knees and examiner feels for crepitus)
- Passive flexion (90 degrees) with internal rotation of hip

SPINE

- "Open your mouth and put 3 of your (*child's own*) fingers in your mouth"
- Lateral flexion of cervical spine—"Try and touch your shoulder with your ear"
- Observe the spine from behind

- "Can you bend and touch your toes?" Observe curve of the spine from side and behind

For further information about the validation of pGALS see: Foster HE, Kay LJ, Friswell M, Coady D, Myers A. Musculoskeletal screening examination (pGALS) for school-age children based on the adult GALS screen. Arthritis Care Research 2006; 55(5); 709–716.

Checklist (6965/DVD-PGALS/06-1)

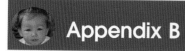

DEVELOPMENT

1. *Gross motor:*
   - Good head control (3 mo)→sitting with support (5 mo)→crawling (9 mo)→cruising (10–11 mo) → unsteady walking (12 mo)→walking alone confidently (15 mo)→run stiffly and walking stairs with one hand held (18 mo)→running well and walking up and down stairs (24 mo) →climb stairs in alternating foot (30 mo)→rides tricycle, stand momentarily on one foot (36 mo)→hops on one foot (48 mo)→skips (60 mo)

2. *Fine motor and adaptive*
   Blocks-books and crayon-beads

   - Open their hand to grasp adult finger (1 mo)→hand mouthing, hold rattle briefly before dropping it (3 mo) !reaching for object, poking an object with index finger, hand transfer by palmer grasp, putting things into mouth (6 mo) →pincer grasp between finger and thumbs, moves arm up and down (9 mo)→pick up small object by thumb and tip of index finger, i.e. fine pincer, point with index finger, hold crayon with palmer grasp, turn several pages of book, release an object on command, build with a few bricks, hand preference (12 mo)→imitate scribbling to and fro, build a tower of 2 cubes after demonstration (15 mo)→build a tower of 3–4, hold pencil in primitive tripod grasp, imitate strokes, dumping pellets from bottle, delicate pincer (18 mo)→build tower of six or more blocks, turn pages singly, does horizontal strokes, copy a vertical lines (24 mo)→7–9 cube tower, mimic horizontal line (30mo)→tower 10 blocks, can imitate bridge with towers, draw circle, copy cross (36 mo)→copy building patterns of three steps using 6 cubes, hold pen in adult fashion, copy square, draw a man, able to thread small beads (48 mo)→copy a triangle, can appreciate heavy and light, draw man with mouth eye, hand leg etc., jigsaw puzzle with interlocking pieces (60 mo).

3. *Language and cognitive*
   Books (naming, color, counting, reasoning, expression, pointing)

   - Laugh and vocalise, smile in response to speech (3 mo)→babbles, squeal in delight, turn to mothers voice or main carers voice (6 mo), object permanence (watch a toy being hidden and then look for it), understands and obeys no (6mo)→use mamma dada, using simple instructions like–come to daddy, clap hands, and wave bye-bye, speak 2–6 recognisable words (12 mo) →understand the names of various parts of the body, identify pictures, understand no, show me, look (15 mo)→know the names of body and point to them, 6–40 recognisable words, indicate desire by pointing, refer to themselves by name, enjoy trying to sing (18 mo)→puts 3 word together, up to 200 words, follow simple instructions (24 mo)→know their full name, nursery rhymes, continuously asking question, refers self to I (30 mo)→knows age/sex, count up to ten, (36 mo)→counting up to 20,tell long story, can say full address (48 mo)→knows name, age, address, birthday, try to write their own name, love to be read stories, names 4 colors (60 mo).

4. *Social and emotional*

Play (solitary, parallel, interactive, competitive)

- Social smile, gaze to adults face when feeding (1 mo)→enjoys bath, stay awake for longer time (3 mo)→feeding with fingers, stranger anxiety, enjoys playing (6 mo)→enjoy songs, needs to have a comfort object, enjoy making noises, can drink from cup (9 mo)→respond to their names, play pat a cake wave good bye both spontaneously and on request, helps getting dressed (12 mo)→casting, i.e. repeatedly throw objects to the floor in play or rejection, carry dolls by their limbs, hair, clothing (15 mo)→feeds self, kisses parent with puckering, solitary play, indicate toilet needs (18 mo)→handles spoon well, help to undress listen to stories, temper tantrums (24 mo)→pretend play, helps put things, dry through nights, may go to toilet independently, play more with children but not sharing, (30 mo)→show affection to siblings, aware of being male/female, take turn in play and enjoy sharing, develop fear, make friends (36 mo)→eat with spoon and fork, wash and dry their hands, undress and dress themselves but cannot do laces, ties or back buttons, shows sensitivity to others (48 mo)→definite likes and dislikes loves to watch a book or video, show sympathy to others, enjoy caring for pets, choose own friends (60 mo)

Vision Development

A baby's eyes are relatively well developed compared to other parts of the body. Vision develops from birth to 7 yr. An approximate guide to ability is:

- Birth: Look, focus on close objects, i.e face
- 2 weeks: Begin to recognise parents
- 4–6 week: starts to smile
- 6 week: Follows brightly coloured target at 20 cm.
- 6 months: Can see across the room.

Vision Testing

- 0–6 months: Observations, fixing, following.
- 6 month to 2 years: Preferential looking, ability to pick up raisins (nonverbal children)
- 2–4 yr: Picture recognition/letter matching
- 4/5 yr + : Normal adult type test

Routine eye test done on all babies born before 32 wk or less than 1500 gm

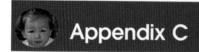

BODY MAP

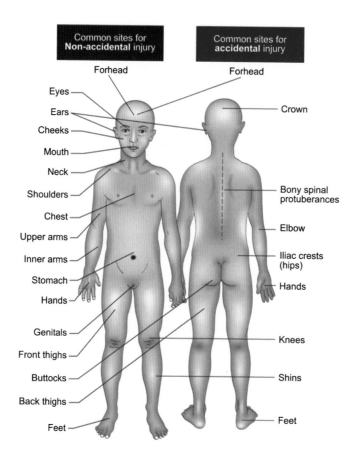

TERMS AND NOMENCLATURE

- F1—Foundation year 1 (pre registration year)
- F2—Foundation year 2
- ST1—ST3: Specialist trainee years 1 to 3 – generally 1st on call
- ST4—ST6: Specialist trainee – 2nd on call (Post MRCPCH)
- Primary care provided by general practitioner (GP)
- DGH—District general hospital
- Tertiary Hospital/Unit—Supraregional centres
- NHS—National Health Service
- NICE—National Institute of clinical excellence

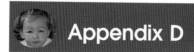

Appendix D

LOCAL AUTHORITY SERVICES FOR CHILDREN IN NEED

Who are 'Children in Need'

Children in need are defined in law as children who are aged under 18 and
- need local authority services to achieve or maintain a reasonable standard of health or development
- need local authority services to prevent significant or further harm to health or development
- are disabled.

The local authority must keep a register of children with disabilities in its area but does not have to keep a register of all children in need.

What Services can the Local Authority Provide

The local authority can provide a range of services for children in need. These can include:
- day care facilities for children under 5 and not yet at school
- after-school and holiday care or activities for school age children
- advice, guidance and counselling
- occupational, social, cultural or recreational activities
- home helps and laundry facilities
- assistance with travelling to and from home in order to use any services provided by the local authority
- assistance for the child and family to have a holiday
- family centres
- financial assistance usually in the form of a loan, see below
- respite care
- looking after the child, see below.

The local authority can also provide the following services to all children in its area, not just children in need:
- day care facilities for children under five and not yet at school
- after-school and holiday care or activities for school age children.

In England, if a child is staying for at least three months away from family in a place of care, at for example a:
- NHS hospital
- Residential school
- Care home
- Independent hospital

The local authority may be able to provide the following services:
- Advice, guidance, counselling
- Family visits to the place of care
- Visits home

In addition to the above services, the local authority, or in Northern Ireland, a local Health and Social Services Trust, has a duty to provide services it considers appropriate for the following children:
- Disabled children
- Children who might otherwise be made subject to care proceedings
- Children who are likely to be involved in crime.

In England, from 1 April 2011, local authorities must provide breaks from caring (respite care) for the parents of disabled children.
- Help to organise a holiday for family members to be together.

http://www.adviceguide.org.uk/index/your_family/family_index_ew/local_authority_services_for_children_in_need.htm